T0292980

Inference Principles for Biostatisticians

Chapman & Hall/CRC Biostatistics Series

Published Titles

Chapman & Hall/CRC Biostatistics Series

Inference Principles for Biostatisticians

Ian C. Marschner

Macquarie University

Australia

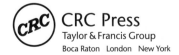

CRC Press
Taylor & Francis Group
Boca Raton London New York

CRC Press is an imprint of the
Taylor & Francis Group, an **informa** business

A CHAPMAN & HALL BOOK

CRC Press
Taylor & Francis Group
6000 Broken Sound Parkway NW, Suite 300
Boca Raton, FL 33487-2742

Printed on acid-free paper
Version Date: 20141024

International Standard Book Number-13: 978-1-4822-2223-4 (Hardback)

Visit the Taylor & Francis Web site at
http://www.taylorandfrancis.com

and the CRC Press Web site at
http://www.crcpress.com

To my family
Simone, Monique, Owen and Eloise.

Contents

Preface

Statistical inference is the science of drawing conclusions on the basis of information that is subject to randomness. Biostatistics is the discipline that underpins the use of statistical inference in the health and medical sciences. This book presents the principles of statistical inference from a biostatistical perspective.

The book is intended for students training to become biostatisticians, or as a background reference for practising biostatisticians. While much of the content is common to other areas of statistics, it is presented from the perspective of a biostatistician, with examples and exercises having a biostatistical flavour. The intention is to provide a sense of context to the theoretical and conceptual foundations of biostatistics.

For over a decade the material in this book has been used as the basis for a one-semester foundation unit in a Master of Biostatistics program, delivered by a consortium of universities under the banner of the Biostatistics Collaboration of Australia. The material provides theoretical underpinnings for subsequent units dealing with core methodologies such as linear models, generalised linear models, survival analysis, longitudinal methods and randomised trials. Thus, the intention in writing this book is not to provide a comprehensive review of biostatistical methods, but rather to lay the conceptual foundation that will prepare the reader for gaining a rigorous understanding of such methods.

As well as presenting the core principles of statistical inference, the book has some noteworthy features. Many extended examples are included, each of which illustrates the key concepts in some depth using a specific biostatistical context. Simulation is used in both the presentation and the exercises, particularly to reinforce the repeated sampling interpretation of many statistical concepts. Simple functions for conducting such simulation studies are provided using the R computing environment. The intention is to suppress the computational complexities in favour of the conceptual lessons.

The book will be most useful for graduate biostatistics programs having broad entry criteria, where students with diverse backgrounds require a solid foundation in the principles of statistical inference. Accordingly, the assumed prior knowledge for the book is not extensive, but it does require mathematical aptitude and prior exposure to basic mathematical and statistical concepts. In particular, the prerequisites for this book are: (i) a basic mathematical background including matrices and calculus; (ii) an introduction to probability concepts including distributions and random variables; and (iii) an introduction to basic statistical concepts including descriptive statistics, confidence intervals and hypothesis testing for means and proportions in one- and two-sample contexts. Some of this prerequisite material is reviewed and used as examples in the book, but the intention is to reinforce and build on prior exposure rather than to present it for the first time. For example, although probability concepts are reviewed and standard methods such as t-tests are used, some prior exposure to this material would be expected.

I would like to thank my colleagues in the Biostatistics Collaboration of Australia, who have created a successful national consortium for training a new generation of biostatisticians in Australia. I would particularly like to thank John Carlin, who played an important role in the initial development of this material, as well as those who have helped to further develop and deliver the material in the years that followed, particularly Patrick Kelly, Adrienne Kirby, Liz Barnes, Rachel O'Connell and all of my colleagues in the Biostatistics Group at the NHMRC Clinical Trials Centre. And finally, I thank the many students who have studied this material, particularly for their feedback that has helped to improve it.

Overall, my primary hope with this book is that mathematically adept students from diverse backgrounds across the health, medical, social and mathematical sciences can be provided with a common foundation on which to subsequently develop a rigorous understanding of biostatistical methodology.

Ian C. Marschner
Sydney, Australia

About the author

Ian Marschner is Head of the Department of Statistics and Professor of Statistics at Macquarie University. He is also Professor of Biostatistics at the University of Sydney, in the National Health and Medical Research Council (NHMRC) Clinical Trials Centre. He has over 25 years of experience as a biostatistician working on health and medical research, particularly involving clinical trials and epidemiological studies of cardiovascular disease, cancer and HIV/AIDS. Formerly he was Director of the Asia Biometrics Centre with the pharmaceutical company Pfizer and was Associate Professor of Biostatistics at Harvard University.

1

Probability and random samples

This chapter introduces the basic inference principle that information about a population can be obtained using a sample from that population. After discussing the concepts of population and sample we interpret this principle in the context of biostatistics, where the goal is typically to understand and improve the health of a population. The importance of using samples that are representative of the population is discussed, which requires the notion of random sampling and the concept of probability. Key probability concepts are then reviewed, including the relative frequency interpretation that forms the basis of the standard approach to statistical inference. We review the common ways of obtaining samples in biostatistics, including prospective, retrospective and cross-sectional samples, and discuss the concepts of sampling variation and bias. Two of the most important measures of population health, risk and prevalence, are defined in terms of probability and are used to illustrate random sampling concepts throughout the chapter.

1.1 Statistical inference

An inference is a conclusion that has been reached on the basis of information or evidence. The term statistical inference refers to a particular type of inferential process, namely, the mathematical science of drawing conclusions using information that is subject to randomness. Two central concepts in statistical inference are the concepts of **population** and **sample**. The basic principle of statistical inference is that conclusions about a population of interest can be made using information contained in a sample from that population.

For now it will be helpful to think of the population as a population in the literal sense, that is, as a complete collection of people or objects of particular interest. Likewise, we can think of the sample as a smaller part of the complete population. In this context, the typical rationale for using a smaller sample to make inferences about a larger population is that the population may be too large to study in its entirety. Later, we will discuss the fact that the population may not always be a literal population, and the sample may not literally be a small part of some larger population. This will mean that the concepts of population and sample sometimes require a broader interpretation. However, for now, these literal meanings of the words population and sample provide a helpful intuitive basis by which to introduce the key concepts of statistical inference.

There are a variety of inferences that could be made about a population using a sample from that population. For example, we may wish to provide a numerical estimate of some important quantity associated with the population, such as the percentage of people that have a particular attribute. Alternatively, we may wish to assess the plausibility of a particular theory or hypothesis about the population. The key issue is that we are using the information in our sample as evidence by which to draw a certain conclusion about the population.

Biostatistics, also sometimes called **medical statistics**, is the discipline that uses statistical inference to study medicine and population health. Thus, in biostatistics the sample usually consists of people drawn from a particular population of interest, and we use the characteristics and health experiences of the people in our sample to infer things about the wider population. This may involve obtaining information about the population, such as measuring the extent of disease or estimating a particular characteristic of the population, such as the average cholesterol level. Or, it may involve understanding how best to intervene to improve health, such as by assessing whether a cholesterol-lowering treatment can improve the health of the population by reducing the occurrence of heart disease.

The fundamental requirement of statistical inference is that the sample is representative of the population. Otherwise, extrapolations from the sample to the population will not be valid. This representativeness is best achieved by choosing the people in our sample using a chance mechanism, and leads to the notion of a random sample. In view of the randomness inherent in our sample, statistical inference therefore involves describing the characteristics of the population using the concept of probability. This means that probability is central to an understanding of statistical inference.

In the remainder of this chapter we will review the main probabilistic concepts used in this book, and then use them to discuss the concept of a random sample in greater detail. Our discussion of probability concepts may at times seem to take us some way away from our central interest of using a random sample to make inferences about a population. However, the probabilistic concepts introduced here will be necessary in subsequent chapters when we study the precise manner in which a random sample can be used to make inferences about a population of interest.

1.2 Probability

When we take a sample from a population using a chance mechanism, the result of our sampling process will involve uncertainty or variability. We will use the term **outcome** to refer to a given realisation of this sampling process. Thus, the variability in our sampling process means that there are various possible outcomes that could occur when we obtain a sample. The set of all possible outcomes is referred to as the **sample space**. Outcomes and sample spaces are the basic elements of interest in the study of probability, the former referring to one possible sample and the latter referring to all possible samples.

For example, suppose our sample consists of two individuals for whom we record whether or not a particular infection is present or absent. For each individual we will denote presence or absence of the infection by 1 and 0, respectively. Then one possible outcome of the sampling process is that both individuals sampled have the infection present, which is an outcome denoted by the pair of infection statuses $(1,1)$. The sample space is the set of all possible outcomes, that is, all possible pairs of infection statuses for the two individuals $\{(0,0),(0,1),(1,0),(1,1)\}$.

A subset of outcomes in the sample space is called an **event**. An event can be interpreted as an observation that could occur in our sample, and each possible event will have a probability assigned to it reflecting the "chance" that the event will actually occur. In our earlier example, consider the event "there is exactly one infected individual in the sample". Two of the outcomes in the sample space correspond to exactly one infected individual, $(0,1)$ and $(1,0)$. The event is therefore denoted by the subset of the sample space $\{(0,1),(1,0)\}$.

Note that events need not correspond to more than one outcome. For example, the event "there are two infected individuals in the sample" consists of just one outcome $\{(1,1)\}$. Indeed, for technical reasons we even allow for impossible events that do not contain any outcomes, such as the event "there are three infected individuals in the sample". In this case the event is denoted by the empty set ϕ.

Since events are defined mathematically as sets, we can use the operations of set intersection $\cap$ and set union $\cup$ to construct new events from existing events. If we consider two events $\mathcal{E}_1$ and $\mathcal{E}_2$, then the new event $\mathcal{E}_1 \cap \mathcal{E}_2$ is interpreted as the event that both $\mathcal{E}_1$ and $\mathcal{E}_2$ occur. Likewise, the new event $\mathcal{E}_1 \cup \mathcal{E}_2$ is interpreted as the event that either $\mathcal{E}_1$ or $\mathcal{E}_2$ or both occur. If the event $\mathcal{E}_1 \cap \mathcal{E}_2$ is the empty set ϕ, then $\mathcal{E}_1$ and $\mathcal{E}_2$ are called **mutually exclusive** events with the interpretation that the two events cannot both occur. For example, the event "either 1 or 2 individuals in the sample are infected" corresponds to the event union

$$\{(0,1),(1,0)\} \cup \{(1,1)\} = \{(0,1),(1,0),(1,1)\}.$$

On the other hand, the event "both 1 and 2 individuals in the sample are infected " corresponds to the event intersection

$$\{(0,1),(1,0)\} \cap \{(1,1)\} = \phi$$

which is impossible since these events are mutually exclusive.

The **probability** assigned to an event is a numerical quantification of the tendency for that event to occur. This means that probability is a function of events, or a function of subsets of the sample space. Consider any event $\mathcal{E}$ that is a subset of the sample space $\mathcal{S}$. Then $\Pr(\mathcal{E})$ denotes the probability that event $\mathcal{E}$ will occur. The function "Pr" is allowed to be any function of subsets of the sample space that satisfies certain requirements that make it a valid probability. Any valid probability must satisfy the following intuitively natural requirements:

1. The probability of any event $\mathscr{E}$ is a number between 0 and 1 inclusive. That is,

$$0 \leq \Pr(\mathscr{E}) \leq 1.$$

2. The probability of a certain event is 1 and the probability of an impossible event is 0. That is,

$$\Pr(\mathscr{S}) = 1 \qquad \text{and} \qquad \Pr(\phi) = 0.$$

3. If two events $\mathscr{E}_1$ and $\mathscr{E}_2$ are mutually exclusive, so they cannot both occur, the probability that either event occurs is the sum of their respective probabilities. That is,

$$\text{if} \quad \mathscr{E}_1 \cap \mathscr{E}_2 = \phi \quad \text{then} \quad \Pr(\mathscr{E}_1 \cup \mathscr{E}_2) = \Pr(\mathscr{E}_1) + \Pr(\mathscr{E}_2).$$

Strictly speaking there are some additional technical complexities associated with the definition of a valid probability which we briefly note for completeness, but which will not affect our subsequent discussions. Firstly, note that the above requirements can actually be expressed more succinctly. For example, the second part of requirement 2 is an implication of the first part. Thus, the requirements of a valid probability, called the **axioms of probability**, are usually written in a slightly briefer but essentially equivalent form to the requirements described above. Secondly, although we have said that probability is a function of subsets of the sample space, we have not said whether a valid probability can be applied to every subset of the sample space, or whether it is restricted to particular subsets of the sample space. In fact, for technical reasons that are beyond our scope here, it is sometimes not possible to define probability for all subsets of the sample space and a complete definition of a probability requires a statement of the collection of subsets of the sample space that we are prepared to apply the probability to. If we call this collection $\mathscr{F}$, then the probability Pr is a function from $\mathscr{F}$ to $[0, 1]$. For our purposes, however, we will suppress this technicality and simply think of the probability Pr as any function that takes subsets of the sample space as an input and gives a number between 0 and 1 as an output, while also satisfying the other requirements described above.

Example 1.1 Consider the example introduced earlier in this section in which a sample of two individuals is taken and an infection status is recorded for each individual. In this case, the sample space $\mathscr{S}$ includes four outcomes, $\mathscr{S} = \{(0,0), (0,1), (1,0), (1,1)\}$. Including the trivial null event ϕ, there are 16 events associated with this sample space, each of which is listed in Table 1.1. Also listed are three potential ways to assign probabilities to each of these events. In each case it can be seen that requirements 1 and 2 are satisfied. However, observe that requirement 3 is not satisfied for the third potential probability assignment, because

$$\Pr(\mathscr{S}) = \Pr(\{(0,0), (0,1), (1,0), (1,1)\}) = 1$$
$$\neq \Pr(\{(0,0)\}) + \Pr(\{(0,1)\}) + \Pr(\{(1,0)\}) + \Pr(\{(1,1)\}) = 1.2.$$

Thus, this assignment of probabilities is invalid. The other two ways of assigning

TABLE 1.1
Three probability assignments to events associated with a sample of
two individuals with sample space $\mathscr{S} = \{(0,0),(0,1),(1,0),(1,1)\}$

Event	probability 1	probability 2	probability 3
ϕ	0	0	0
$\{(0,0)\}$	0.9025	0.3025	0.3000
$\{(0,1)\}$	0.0475	0.2475	0.3000
$\{(1,0)\}$	0.0475	0.2475	0.3000
$\{(1,1)\}$	0.0025	0.2025	0.3000
$\{(0,0),(0,1)\}$	0.9500	0.5500	0.6000
$\{(0,0),(1,0)\}$	0.9500	0.5500	0.6000
$\{(0,0),(1,1)\}$	0.9050	0.5050	0.6000
$\{(0,1),(1,0)\}$	0.0950	0.4950	0.6000
$\{(0,1),(1,1)\}$	0.0500	0.4500	0.6000
$\{(1,0),(1,1)\}$	0.0500	0.4500	0.6000
$\{(0,0),(0,1),(1,0)\}$	0.9975	0.7975	0.9000
$\{(0,0),(0,1),(1,1)\}$	0.9525	0.7525	0.9000
$\{(0,0),(1,0),(1,1)\}$	0.9525	0.7525	0.9000
$\{(0,1),(1,0),(1,1)\}$	0.0975	0.6975	0.9000
$\mathscr{S}$	1	1	1

probabilities do satisfy requirement 3, so these are both valid. Even though they are
both valid, notice that they are quite different in terms of the actual probabilities that
they assign to the different events.

While the probability axioms specify a collection of minimal requirements that
any valid probability must satisfy, many other implications follow from these basic
requirements. For example, a very important property that follows from the axioms
is

$$\Pr(\mathscr{E}_1 \cup \mathscr{E}_2) = \Pr(\mathscr{E}_1) + \Pr(\mathscr{E}_2) - \Pr(\mathscr{E}_1 \cap \mathscr{E}_2).$$

It can be seen that this property is a generalisation of requirement 3 to the situation
where the two events are not necessarily mutually exclusive. For example, suppose
event $\mathscr{E}_1$ is "exactly one individual is infected" and event $\mathscr{E}_2$ is "the first individual
is infected". Then $\mathscr{E}_1 = \{(0,1),(1,0)\}$, $\mathscr{E}_2 = \{(1,0),(1,1)\}$ and $\mathscr{E}_1 \cap \mathscr{E}_2 = \{(1,0)\}$.
Thus, using the two valid probability assignments from Table 1.1, the above property
implies, respectively, that $\Pr(\mathscr{E}_1 \cup \mathscr{E}_2) = \Pr(\{(0,1),(1,0),(1,1)\})$ is

$$0.0950 + 0.0500 - 0.0475 = 0.0975 \quad \text{and} \quad 0.4950 + 0.4500 - 0.2475 = 0.6975.$$

Notice that in each case the probability calculation concords with the probability
assigned to the event $\{(0,1),(1,0),(1,1)\}$ in Table 1.1.

1.3   Relative frequency

The above discussion is an abstract mathematical description of probability as a function of subsets of a sample space, but it does not give us much intuition into what probability actually is. From a statistical point of view we need to go further and associate an interpretation to the numerical value that quantifies the probability of an event. The most common such interpretation used in statistics is called the **relative frequency** interpretation, and leads to the **frequentist** school of statistical inference.

Consider N samples taken in an identical fashion from the population. We will refer to such a collection as N repeated samples. Now consider a particular event that could, or could not, occur in each of these N repeated samples. If we let f_N be the number of samples in which the event did occur, then f_N is referred to as the frequency of the event, and f_N/N is referred to as the relative frequency of the event. Thus, the relative frequency of the event is simply the proportion of times that the event occurred in the N repeated samples.

Under the relative frequency interpretation of probability, the probability of an event is interpreted as the proportion of times this event would occur in a long sequence of repeated samples. That is, probability is interpreted as the limiting value of the relative frequency of the event as the number of repeated samples gets larger and larger,

$$\text{probability} = \lim_{N \to \infty} \left(\frac{f_N}{N} \right).$$

For example, consider the event discussed earlier that there is exactly one infected individual in a sample of two individuals. Then a probability of 0.1 for this event means that in a large number of repeated samples of two individuals, 10% of such repeated samples will have exactly one individual infected. Importantly, this means that to interpret the probability of an event occurring in a single sample, we need to think about what would happen in a large number of repeated samples.

For most of this book we will restrict ourselves to this relative frequency interpretation of probability, which in turn means that the statistical inference principles that we discuss are from the frequentist school of statistical inference. This is the most common type of statistical inference in practice, but it is not the only type. Other interpretations of probability can lead to different types of statistical inference principles. In Chapter 7 we will discuss a different interpretation of probability that leads to the so-called Bayesian school of statistical inference.

Example 1.2 One of the most important examples of the use of probability in biostatistics is for quantifying **risk**. An individual's risk of an event is defined as the probability of the individual experiencing the event within a specific time frame. This means that risk is always expressed with reference to a specific period of time. For example, consider an individual arriving at the emergency room of a hospital with a heart attack. It is natural to consider the risk of death for this individual, which means the probability of death within a specific time frame. Suppose we say that the risk of death within one month of the heart attack is 15%. To interpret what we mean by this statement we can use the relative frequency interpretation of probability. Under this interpretation we need to think about what would happen if we observed N individuals from the same population who arrived at the emergency room having a heart attack. If we observed these N individuals for the month following their heart attack and obtained the relative frequency of death, in other words the proportion who died within one month, then a probability of 15% means that the relative frequency will approach the value 15% as N increases towards infinity. Of course, for small N the relative frequency may be different to 15%, either higher or lower, but as N increases we would expect it to oscillate more tightly, and the value that it finally settles at is interpreted as the probability of the event. Figure 1.1 displays a simulation that illustrates the dependence of the relative frequency of death on the number of individuals observed, and the limiting value of this relative frequency corresponding to the risk of death. Importantly, in order to interpret the risk of death for a single individual, we have had to think about the occurrence of death in a large number of individuals presenting to the hospital with a heart attack.

1.4 Probability distributions

A **random variable** is a function of outcomes in the sample space. It can be thought of as an uncertain quantity that can be observed as a result of taking our sample, and which takes on values with particular probabilities. If a random variable can take on only a discrete set of values then it is referred to as a **discrete random variable**, whereas if the values that a random variable can take on form a continuum then it is referred to as a **continuous random variable**. For example, the gender of a randomly sampled individual is discrete while their cholesterol level is continuous.

Statements about a random variable taking on a particular value or having a value in a particular range are events. We can therefore assign probabilities to such events. For example, for a random variable X and a given number x, statements such as $X = x$ and $X \leq x$ are events. We can therefore assign probabilities $\Pr(X = x)$ and $\Pr(X \leq x)$ to such events. A general convention is that random variables are denoted by upper-case letters, while the values that they can take on are denoted by lower-case letters. The distinction between an upper-case random variable and a lower-case random variable value will be important in subsequent chapters. It can be thought of as the distinction between a function and a particular value that a function takes on.

The **probability distribution** for a random variable is a rule for assigning a probability to any event stating that the random variable takes on a specific value or lies in a specific range. There are various ways to specify the probability distribution of a random variable. One way we will use is the **cumulative distribution function**. The

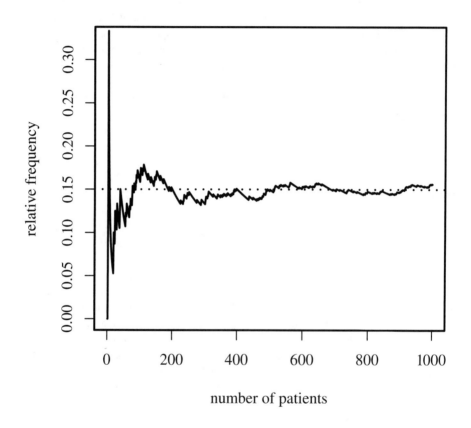

FIGURE 1.1
Relative frequency of death within one month of a heart attack with increasing sample size. Dotted line is the population risk of death

cumulative distribution function of a random variable X is a function $F_X(x)$ such that

$$F_X(x) = \Pr(X \leq x)$$

for any number x. Any valid cumulative distribution function must therefore satisfy the following three properties:

(i) $\lim_{x \to \infty} F_X(x) = 1$ (ii) $\lim_{x \to -\infty} F_X(x) = 0$ (iii) $F_X(x_1) \geq F_X(x_2)$ if $x_1 \geq x_2$.

There are two additional functions of central importance in specifying the probability distribution of a random variable, one for discrete random variables and the other for continuous random variables.

The **probability function** associated with a discrete random variable X is a function that gives the probability that the random variable will equal any specific value. That is, the probability function is

$$f_X(x) = \Pr(X = x)$$

where x is any number in the set of possible values that X can take on. For any discrete random variable, $\sum_x f_X(x) = 1$, where the summation is taken over all possible values that X can take on.

The **probability density function** associated with a continuous random variable is the derivative of the cumulative distribution function

$$f_X(x) = \frac{d}{dx} F_X(x).$$

It specifies the probability that a continuous random variable will fall into any given range through the relationship

$$\Pr(l \leq X \leq u) = \int_l^u f_X(x)dx$$

and must therefore always integrate to 1 over the range $(-\infty, \infty)$. Note that the probability density function does not give the probability that a continuous random variable is equal to a specific value. For a continuous random variable it is always the case that $\Pr(X = x) = 0$.

The probability distribution of a random variable has various attributes that summarise the way the random variable tends to behave. The **expectation**, or **mean**, of a random variable is the average value that the random variable takes on. For discrete random variables the expectation is given by

$$E(X) = \sum_x x f_X(x)$$

where the summation is over all possible values that the random variable X can take on. For continuous random variables the expectation is given by

$$E(X) = \int_{-\infty}^{\infty} x f_X(x)dx.$$

These two expressions for the expectation of a random variable are sometimes written in a unified fashion using integration with respect to the cumulative distribution function, which allows the expectation of both discrete and continuous random variables to be given by the same expression,

$$E(X) = \int_{-\infty}^{\infty} x dF_X(x).$$

This unified form will be used in Chapter 8, where it will be interpreted as the summation form of expectation when the distribution is discrete with probability function $f_X(x)$, and will be interpreted as the integral form of expectation when the distribution is continuous with probability density function $f_X(x)$.

Since the sum or integral of a linear function yields a linear function of the sum or integral, expectations possess an important linearity property, which is that for constants c_0 and c_1

$$E(c_0 + c_1 X) = c_0 + c_1 E(X).$$

The **variance** of a random variable is a measure of the degree of variation that a random variable exhibits. It is defined as

$$\text{Var}(X) = E\left[(X - E(X))^2\right] = E(X^2) - E(X)^2$$

for both continuous and discrete random variables. Unlike expectations, the linearity property does not hold for variances, but is replaced by the equally important property

$$\text{Var}(c_0 + c_1 X) = c_1^2 \text{Var}(X).$$

Another important aspect of probability distributions are **percentiles**. For $\alpha \in (0,1)$, we will call the α-percentile of a probability distribution the point below which $100\alpha\%$ of the distribution falls. This means that a random variable with that probability distribution has probability α of taking a value below the α-percentile. More specifically, the α-percentile of a probability distribution with cumulative distribution function $F_X(x)$ is the point p_α that satisfies $F_X(p_\alpha) = \alpha$. For example, the 0.5 percentile, called the **median**, is the point below which half of the probability distribution lies. Similarly, the 0.25 and 0.75 percentiles, called **quartiles**, specify the points below which one-quarter and three-quarters of the distribution lies. Other percentiles of a probability distribution will also be of interest, particularly when we come to discuss confidence intervals in subsequent chapters.

In practice, the probability distributions that are commonly used in statistical inference are based on a simple and flexible function for $f_X(x)$ or $F_X(x)$. We will consider two such commonly used probability distributions subsequently in this chapter, the binomial and normal distributions. Other commonly used probability distributions are reviewed in Appendix 1 and will be used elsewhere in this book. Typically the function defining the probability distribution is not fully specified, but rather depends on one or more unspecified fixed quantities, such as the mean or the variance. These quantities are referred to as parameters and are usually interpreted as important characteristics of the population of interest. One of the main tasks of statistical inference is to determine values for these parameters and to assess the plausibility of hypotheses about the parameters. This is considered in detail in subsequent chapters.

Example 1.3 In Table 1.1 we specified two valid ways to assign probabilities to the events associated with sampling two individuals and observing their infection status as present or absent. Suppose we now define a random variable T to be the number of infected individuals in the sample. Since the possible values that T can take are simply 0, 1 and 2, T is a discrete random variable. As for any random variable, T is a function of outcomes in the sample space, meaning that for each of the possible outcomes, T will take on a corresponding value. Table 1.2 lists the value of T corresponding to each of the outcomes in the sample space. Also listed in Table 1.2 is a possible probability function $f_T(t)$ which gives $\Pr(T = t)$ for each possible value of T, along with the corresponding cumulative distribution function $F_T(t)$ which gives $\Pr(T \leq t)$. Since there are only three possible values for T, it is quite manageable to list out $f_T(t)$ and $F_T(t)$ for each value. However, this soon becomes unmanageable if T can take on many values, such as would occur if our sample consisted of 100 individuals. It is therefore useful to have a simple and flexible function that specifies the probability distribution of T. Consider the function

$$f_T(t) = \frac{2!}{(2-t)!t!}0.05^t(1-0.05)^{2-t} \qquad t = 0,1,2$$

which is a special case of the more general function

$$f_T(t) = \frac{n!}{(n-t)!t!}\theta^t(1-\theta)^{n-t} \qquad t = 0,1,\ldots,n$$

with $n = 2$ and $\theta = 0.05$. It may be verified that this probability function yields the probabilities in Table 1.2, as well as the first probability assignment in Table 1.1. This illustrates how an entire probability distribution can be captured with a single function. As reviewed in Appendix 1, this particular probability distribution is known as the binomial distribution, which is often an appropriate distribution for a random variable specifying the number of events that have occurred out of n trials. In this case, we denote this distribution as

$$T \overset{d}{=} \text{Bin}(2,0.05)$$

where the notation $\overset{d}{=}$ means "is distributed as". There is no simple form of $F_T(t)$ for the binomial distribution, so $\Pr(T \leq t)$ would have to be calculated by summing up values of $f_T(t)$, as illustrated in Table 1.2. The expectation and variance for a binomial random variable do have simple forms, which in this case are $E(T) = n\theta = 0.1$ and $\text{Var}(T) = n\theta(1-\theta) = 0.095$. Note that a key assumption for the validity of the binomial distribution is that the results of each trial, that is the infection status of each individual, must be "independent" of each other. The concept of independence is an important probabilistic concept that we will discuss in detail in the next section.

TABLE 1.2
Probability distribution for T, the
number infected in a sample of two
individuals

t	Event $T = t$	$f_T(t)$	$F_T(t)$
0	$\{(0,0)\}$	0.9025	0.9025
1	$\{(0,1),(1,0)\}$	0.0950	0.9975
2	$\{(1,1)\}$	0.0025	1

1.5   Independence

Independence is a property that applies to both events and random variables. The concept of independence requires us to think about how the probability of an event might change once we know that some other event has occurred. This introduces us to conditional probability, which we define first, before considering the concept of independence.

For two events $\mathscr{E}_1$ and $\mathscr{E}_2$, the **conditional probability** that $\mathscr{E}_1$ occurs given that $\mathscr{E}_2$ has occurred is denoted $\Pr(\mathscr{E}_1|\mathscr{E}_2)$ and is defined as

$$\Pr(\mathscr{E}_1|\mathscr{E}_2) = \frac{\Pr(\mathscr{E}_1 \cap \mathscr{E}_2)}{\Pr(\mathscr{E}_2)}.$$

From a mathematical point of view, conditional probability can only be defined for events $\mathscr{E}_2$ that are not impossible, so that $\Pr(\mathscr{E}_2) \neq 0$ in the denominator of the definition. Clearly, this is also an intuitively natural requirement since it does not make sense for us to condition on the occurrence of an impossible event.

With this definition of conditional probability, the two events $\mathscr{E}_1$ and $\mathscr{E}_2$ are said to be **independent events** if

$$\Pr(\mathscr{E}_1|\mathscr{E}_2) = \Pr(\mathscr{E}_1).$$

This can be interpreted as the property that the occurrence of the event $\mathscr{E}_2$ does not affect the probability of occurrence of the event $\mathscr{E}_1$. It is straightforward to verify that the reverse is also true, namely, that the occurrence of the event $\mathscr{E}_1$ does not affect the probability of occurrence of the event $\mathscr{E}_2$.

In view of the conditional probability that appears in the definition of independent events, we can re-express this definition by saying that $\mathscr{E}_1$ and $\mathscr{E}_2$ are independent events if they satisfy the multiplicative property

$$\Pr(\mathscr{E}_1 \cap \mathscr{E}_2) = \Pr(\mathscr{E}_1)\Pr(\mathscr{E}_2).$$

This is the typical way that independence of events is defined, and it has a slight advantage over the earlier definition in terms of conditional probability in that it is applicable even when one of the events has zero probability.

Statistical inference makes more use of the concept of independence when applied to random variables, which can be defined analogously to the way we defined it for events. Consider two random variables X_1 and X_2, with cumulative distribution functions $F_1(x_1)$ and $F_2(x_2)$, respectively. The random variables X_1 and X_2 are said to be **independent random variables** if

$$\Pr(X_1 \le x_1 \mid X_2 \le x_2) = \Pr(X_1 \le x_1) = F_1(x_1)$$

or equivalently

$$\Pr(X_2 \le x_2 \mid X_1 \le x_1) = \Pr(X_2 \le x_2) = F_2(x_2)$$

where x_1 and x_2 are any numbers in the range of possible values of X_1 and X_2, respectively. Thus, loosely speaking, we can say that for two independent random variables, knowing the value of one random variable does not affect the probability distribution of the other.

Similarly to our discussion for independence of events, independence of random variables can be defined using the multiplicative property

$$\Pr(\{X_1 \le x_1\} \cap \{X_2 \le x_2\}) = \Pr(X_1 \le x_1)\Pr(X_2 \le x_2) = F_1(x_1)F_2(x_2).$$

We can see from this form that independence of random variables is defined in terms of independence of the two events $X_1 \le x_1$ and $X_2 \le x_2$.

The above discussion introduces us to the concept of the joint probability distribution of two random variables. Generalising the definition of a probability distribution for a single random variable, the **joint probability distribution** of two random variables is a rule for assigning probabilities to any event stating that the two random variables simultaneously take on specific values or lie in specific ranges. Like the probability distribution of a single random variable, the joint probability distribution can be characterised by various functions. The first of these is a generalisation of the cumulative distribution function. Using the shorthand notation

$$\Pr(X_1 \le x_1, X_2 \le x_2) \equiv \Pr(\{X_1 \le x_1\} \cap \{X_2 \le x_2\})$$

then the **joint cumulative distribution function** of two random variables X_1 and X_2 is the function of two variables

$$F_{X_1,X_2}(x_1,x_2) = \Pr(X_1 \le x_1, X_2 \le x_2).$$

Thus, it can be seen that independence of two random variables is equivalent to their joint cumulative distribution function factoring into the product of their individual cumulative distribution functions.

Analogously to the single random variable context, we can also define the **joint probability function** of two discrete random variables X_1 and X_2 as the function of two variables

$$f_{X_1,X_2}(x_1,x_2) = \Pr(X_1 = x_1, X_2 = x_2).$$

Likewise, we can define the **joint probability density function** of two continuous random variables X_1 and X_2 as the function of two variables that comes from partial differentiation of the joint cumulative distribution function, with respect x_1 and x_2. That is,

$$f_{X_1,X_2}(x_1,x_2) = \frac{\partial}{\partial x_1}\left(\frac{\partial}{\partial x_2}F_{X_1,X_2}(x_1,x_2)\right)$$

where, using standard calculus notation, partial differentiation is denoted using the symbol ∂ in place of the d used in univariate differentiation. The joint probability density function specifies the probability that the two continuous random variables will simultaneously fall into any two given ranges through the relationship

$$\Pr(l_1 \le X_1 \le u_1, l_2 \le X_2 \le u_2) = \int_{l_1}^{u_1}\int_{l_2}^{u_2} f_{X_1,X_2}(x_1,x_2)dx_2dx_1.$$

Although we used the joint cumulative distribution function to define independence of two random variables, independence can equivalently be defined in terms of their joint probability density function or joint probability function. Thus, the multiplicative property for independence of two random variables can equivalently be expressed as

$$f_{X_1,X_2}(x_1,x_2) = f_1(x_1)f_2(x_2)$$

where $f_1(x_1)$ and $f_2(x_2)$ are either the probability density functions or probability functions of X_1 and X_2, respectively, depending on whether they are continuous or discrete random variables.

Another multiplicative property that can exist between two random variables is

$$E(XY) = E(X)E(Y).$$

When this property holds we say that X and Y are **uncorrelated**. Being uncorrelated random variables is a weaker property than being independent random variables, in the sense that independent implies uncorrelated but not vice versa. When $E(XY) \ne E(X)E(Y)$ then the difference is called the covariance of X and Y

$$\mathrm{Cov}(X,Y) = E(XY) - E(X)E(Y) = E\big[(X - E(X))(Y - E(Y))\big].$$

It can be seen that uncorrelated random variables have zero covariance, and that covariance is a generalisation of variance, in the sense that $\mathrm{Cov}(X,X) = \mathrm{Var}(X)$. A measure of the extent to which two random variables depart from being uncorrelated is the **correlation**

$$\mathrm{Corr}(X,Y) = \frac{\mathrm{Cov(X,Y)}}{\sqrt{\mathrm{Var}(X)\mathrm{Var}(Y)}}.$$

The correlation is scaled such that it always lies between -1 and 1, with 0 corresponding to being uncorrelated. It is important in studying the linear relationship between two variables, with the extremes of -1 and 1 corresponding to a perfect negative and positive linear relationship, respectively. Although being uncorrelated implies that there is no linear relationship between two variables, it does not preclude that some other relationship exists. This is why independence is a stronger property than being uncorrelated, since it implies that there is no relationship at all, linear or otherwise.

The main use of the concept of independence in this book is for modelling the probabilistic behaviour of a sample taken at random from a population of interest. In particular, we will often use a collection of n random variables to represent the attributes of n different individuals. In this context, independence means that an observation on one individual does not affect the probability distribution associated with an observation on another individual. Random samples will be discussed in more detail in Section 1.7, however, for now we simply note that the definition of independence of two random variables discussed above extends naturally to independence of a larger collection of n random variables. In particular, n random variables are independent if their joint cumulative distribution function factors into the product of their n individual cumulative distribution functions. That is, extending the notation used for the joint distribution of two random variables, $X = (X_1, \ldots, X_n)$ is an independent collection of random variables if for any vector of numbers $x = (x_1, \ldots, x_n)$

$$F_X(x) = \Pr(X_1 \leq x_1, \ldots, X_n \leq x_n) = \prod_{i=1}^{n} F_i(x_i).$$

For discrete random variables, this definition of independence can equivalently be stated in terms of the joint probability function

$$f_X(x) = \Pr(X_1 = x_1, \ldots, X_n = x_n) = \prod_{i=1}^{n} f_i(x_i).$$

For continuous random variables, it can equivalently be stated in terms of the joint probability density function

$$f_X(x) = \prod_{i=1}^{n} f_i(x_i)$$

where $f_X(x)$ is the derivative of the joint cumulative distribution function, with respect to each of the x_i variables.

We note in passing that the above definition of independence of a collection of random variables is more accurately referred to as **mutual independence**, however, in this book we will not have the need to consider other types of independence and therefore suppress this technicality.

Example 1.4 Recall the random variable T defined in Example 1.3, which is the number infected in a sample of two individuals. Now consider the random variable T_1, which takes the value 1 if the first individual is infected and 0 otherwise. Likewise, we can define the random variable T_2 corresponding to the second individual. Consider the three events $T = 1$, $T_1 = 1$ and $T_2 = 1$, which we denote $\mathscr{E}_0$, $\mathscr{E}_1$ and $\mathscr{E}_2$, respectively. From Table 1.2 we know that $\mathscr{E}_0 = \{(0,1),(1,0)\}$ and $\Pr(\mathscr{E}_0) = 0.095$, based on the first probability assignment from Table 1.1. Likewise we have $\mathscr{E}_1 = \{(1,0),(1,1)\}$ and $\Pr(\mathscr{E}_1) = 0.05$, as well as $\mathscr{E}_2 = \{(0,1),(1,1)\}$ and

$\Pr(\mathscr{E}_2) = 0.05$, again using the first probability assignment from Table 1.1. We can therefore calculate the conditional probability

$$\Pr(\mathscr{E}_1|\mathscr{E}_0) = \frac{\Pr(\mathscr{E}_1 \cap \mathscr{E}_0)}{\Pr(\mathscr{E}_0)} = \frac{\Pr(\{(1,0)\})}{0.095} = \frac{0.0475}{0.095} = 0.5.$$

This result essentially says that, given we know exactly one person is infected, it is equally likely to be individual 1 or 2. Notice that $\mathscr{E}_0$ and $\mathscr{E}_1$ are not independent events since $\Pr(\mathscr{E}_1|\mathscr{E}_0) \neq \Pr(\mathscr{E}_1)$. Intuitively this makes sense, because knowledge that there is one infected individual in the sample should provide information about whether or not individual 1 is infected. On the other hand,

$$\Pr(\mathscr{E}_1 \cap \mathscr{E}_2) = \Pr(\{(1,1)\}) = 0.0025 = 0.05 \times 0.05 = \Pr(\mathscr{E}_1)\Pr(\mathscr{E}_2),$$

showing that the events $T_1 = 1$ and $T_2 = 1$ are independent events. The same process can be followed for any other values of the random variables T_1 and T_2 to show that

$$\Pr(T_1 = t_1, T_2 = t_2) = \Pr(T_1 = t_1)\Pr(T_2 = t_2) \qquad t_1 = 0,1 \quad t_2 = 0,1.$$

In other words, the joint probability function factors into the product of the individual probability functions, so the random variables T_1 and T_2 are independent random variables.

1.6 Normal distribution

We will make use of various probability distributions throughout this book, and Appendix 1 provides a summary of some of the most important distributions. However, there is one distribution that stands out as more important than the others, namely, the **normal distribution**. The importance of the normal distribution arises not so much because biostatistical data tends to follow a normal distribution, but rather because of its general importance in large samples, where it provides a way to unify many of the common statistical inference tools. A discussion of the importance of the normal distribution in large samples is provided in Section 1.10. For now we simply review some of the key features of the normal distribution.

Consider a continuous random variable X with $\mu = E(X)$ and $\sigma^2 = \text{Var}(X)$. We say that X has a normal distribution, written

$$X \stackrel{d}{=} N(\mu, \sigma^2),$$

if the probability density function of X has the form

$$f_X(x) = \frac{1}{\sigma\sqrt{2\pi}} \exp\left\{-\frac{(x-\mu)^2}{2\sigma^2}\right\} \qquad x \in (-\infty, \infty) \quad \mu \in (-\infty, \infty) \quad \sigma > 0.$$

Since $f_X(x)$ depends on μ and σ, the distribution is not fully specified until the values of μ and σ have been specified. As alluded to in Section 1.4, in the context of statistical inference one of the main tasks is to use the sample to estimate μ and σ so that the distribution is fully specified.

Unlike the probability density function $f_X(x)$, the cumulative distribution function $F_X(x)$ is not a convenient function and needs to be calculated numerically from the relationship

$$F_X(x) = \int_{-\infty}^{x} f_X(u)du.$$

This is generally carried out using a special case of the normal distribution, called the **standard normal distribution**, which is the $N(0,1)$ distribution that arises from setting $\mu = 0$ and $\sigma = 1$. If we denote the cumulative distribution function of the standard normal distribution by the function

$$\Phi(x) = \frac{1}{\sqrt{2\pi}} \int_{-\infty}^{x} \exp\left\{-\frac{u^2}{2}\right\} du$$

then the cumulative distribution function associated with any other normal distribution can be calculated using the relationship

$$F_X(x) = \Phi\left(\frac{x-\mu}{\sigma}\right).$$

This means that only the standard normal cumulative distribution function needs to be calculated numerically, and computations associated with any other normal distribution can be expressed in terms of the standard normal distribution. An important calculation associated with the normal distribution is percentile calculation, which we will use in various inference contexts. Using the definition of percentile from Section 1.4, the α-percentile of the standard normal distribution, which we will write as z_α, is the value that satisfies $\Phi(z_\alpha) = \alpha$. Equivalently, it can be expressed as $z_\alpha = \Phi^{-1}(\alpha)$, where Φ^{-1} is the inverse standard normal cumulative distribution function. The percentiles of the standard normal distribution, and their relationship with the percentiles of any other normal distribution, are depicted in Figure 1.2. This figure also illustrates the classic bell shape of the normal probability density function, including its symmetry about the mean.

In Section 1.5 we discussed the joint probability distribution associated with two random variables. One such joint distribution is the **bivariate normal distribution**. Consider two normally distributed random variables $X \overset{d}{=} N(\mu_X, \sigma_X^2)$ and $Y \overset{d}{=} N(\mu_Y, \sigma_Y^2)$, with $\mathrm{Corr}(X,Y) = \rho$ and hence $\mathrm{Cov}(X,Y) = \rho\sigma_X\sigma_Y$. We call μ the mean vector and Σ the variance-covariance matrix where

$$\mu = \begin{bmatrix} \mu_X \\ \mu_Y \end{bmatrix} \quad \text{and} \quad \Sigma = \begin{bmatrix} \sigma_X^2 & \rho\sigma_X\sigma_Y \\ \rho\sigma_X\sigma_Y & \sigma_Y^2 \end{bmatrix}.$$

Then X and Y have a bivariate normal distribution, written

$$\mathbf{X} \overset{d}{=} N_2(\mu, \Sigma) \quad \text{where } \mathbf{X} = \begin{bmatrix} X \\ Y \end{bmatrix}$$

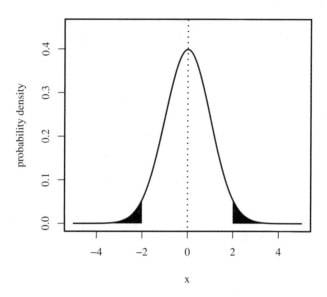

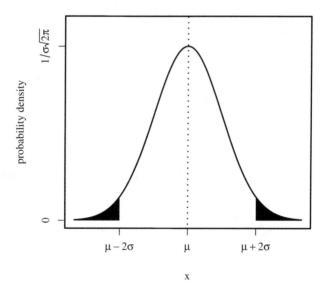

FIGURE 1.2
Probability density functions of the standard normal distribution (top) and $N(\mu, \sigma^2)$
(bottom) distributions. Shaded regions are of equal area $\Phi(-2)$

if their joint probability density function is of the form

$$f_{X,Y}(x,y) = f_{\mathbf{X}}(\mathbf{x}) = \frac{1}{2\pi\sigma_X\sigma_Y\sqrt{1-\rho^2}}\exp\left\{-\frac{1}{2}(\mathbf{x}-\mu)^{\mathrm{T}}\Sigma^{-1}(\mathbf{x}-\mu)\right\}.$$

Although this joint probability density function is most succinctly expressed as a function of $\mathbf{x} = (x,y)$ using vector and matrix notation, the quadratic form inside the exponential function can be expanded, as covered in the exercises, to express the function in terms of x and y. Furthermore, this bivariate normal distribution generalises to the **multivariate normal distribution** for a vector of k random variables $\mathbf{X} = (X_1,\ldots,X_k)^{\mathrm{T}}$, as described in Appendix 1. In this case we write

$$\mathbf{X} \stackrel{d}{=} \mathrm{N}_k(\mu,\Sigma),$$

where μ is a $k \times 1$ mean vector and Σ is a $k \times k$ variance-covariance matrix.

One use of the multivariate normal distribution is for modelling **correlated data**, such as where we have taken multiple observations on the same individual. For example, we may observe cholesterol level and blood pressure on the same individual, or cholesterol level at two different times on the same individual. In each case, the two random variables are likely to be correlated, and the bivariate normal distribution can provide a model for their joint behaviour. Correlated data analysis is a more advanced statistical inference topic that is beyond our scope in this book, so we will not make use of the multivariate normal distribution for this purpose. Another use of the multivariate normal distribution is to model the large sample behaviour of two or more random variables calculated from our sample and which are used to estimate important characteristics of our population. We will return to this in detail when we discuss estimation methods in Chapter 4, which will build on our discussion in Section 1.10 of the importance of the normal distribution in large samples.

1.7 Random samples

In order to use a sample for making inferences about a population, the sample must in some sense be representative of the population. This is achieved by choosing individuals from the population at random. This means that each individual in the population will have a certain probability of being included in the sample. The basic requirement of a random sample, sometimes called a **simple random sample**, is that all individuals in the population have the same probability of being included in the sample. This ensures that the sample is representative of the population and can be used to make inferences about the population. When combined with independence of individuals we will call the sample an **independent random sample**, and this will be the primary object of study in this book. In biostatistics, our sample often involves a collection of individuals whose health experiences can be assumed to be independent of each other, meaning that independent random samples are often encountered in biostatistics. However, it should be noted that more complicated random sampling processes can sometimes be used, and we will touch on the nature and validity of these in the next section.

The way in which a random sample is obtained from a population is a very important element of statistical inference. In this book, our primary focus is on the statistical principles that are used to make inferences once we have a sample from a population, rather than a detailed study of the processes by which samples are obtained. Nonetheless, it is helpful for us to have in mind an understanding of the most common ways that samples are obtained in biostatistics. Broadly speaking, we can classify commonly used biostatistical sampling processes into three main types. Each type of sample involves identifying a random sample of individuals from the population, but they differ in the way that information is collected about the individuals.

The first type of sample is a **prospective sample**. In prospective samples, the individuals in our sample are observed over time and information is collected about their health experiences during the period of observation. Thus, prospective samples begin with sampling at a certain point in time, and involve observation of individuals forward in time. The second type of sample is a **retrospective sample**. In retrospective samples, information about the individuals' history is collected, but unlike prospective studies, no further observation into the future is conducted. Thus, retrospective samples begin with sampling at a certain point in time, and effectively involve observation of individuals backward in time. The third type of sample is a **cross-sectional sample**. In cross-sectional samples, information about the individuals' current situation is collected, but no observation forward or backward in time is conducted. Thus, cross-sectional samples are limited to providing a snapshot of the current status of the population.

Further classification of sampling types beyond these basic types may also occur, depending on the objective of the particular study. In particular, prospective samples may be further classified by whether they are **observational** or **interventional**. As the name suggests, prospective observational samples, which are also called **cohort studies**, simply involve observing information about the experiences of the cohort of individuals in our sample, without intervening to try to improve things. Interventional samples, on the other hand, involve the study of interventions that could improve the health of the population, and lead to further complexities such as how the intervention should be implemented in our sample. Throughout this book we will use the different types of samples to introduce inferential concepts, and we will sometimes take the opportunity to consider their features in more depth, albeit without attempting a comprehensive discussion of study design. For example, the extended example of Chapter 5 provides further discussion of some of the concepts behind interventional studies, including the concept of randomisation.

The above discussion introduces us to the diversity and complexity of sampling types that can occur in practice, and each of the sampling types have their own advantages and disadvantages. For example, retrospective and cross-sectional samples tend to be easier and quicker to obtain because there is no requirement to observe individuals over time. On the other hand, prospective samples tend to be more informative and less susceptible to the sorts of biases that we will discuss in the next section. The pros and cons of different types of random samples are of major importance in biostatistics, coming under the general area of **study design**. From our point of view in this book, however, the primary importance of sample type will be that it determines the type of statistical model that we use as the basis of our statistical inferences. The concept of a statistical model, which uses the notion of probability to describe the randomness in our sample, will be illustrated below and will form the foundation of our discussion of inference concepts beginning in the next chapter.

The observations that we make based on our sample are generically referred to as the **data**. It is the data that provide the information by which we can make our inferences about the population. As we have discussed, we will typically think of the data as having been generated by identifying a sample of individuals from a large population of interest and observing certain attributes of these individuals, using the types of sampling processes discussed above. While this is quite common in biostatistics, there are other ways that a random sample can be obtained. Indeed, in some contexts our sample may not literally arise from a random sampling process, but it may still be reasonable to view the data as having been randomly sampled. For example, routine health surveillance may involve the recording of all diagnoses of a disease in a particular population, without any literal process of random sampling. Nonetheless, statistical inference can still be used by viewing the data as a random realisation from among the "population" of all possible disease diagnoses that could have arisen. In this case the random sampling process involves a more idealised **data generating mechanism**, and we would need to use probability to model the randomness in this mechanism. Thus, while it is usually most intuitive to think about statistical inference in terms of random sampling from a literal population, sometimes a broader interpretation of a random sample is required. As we discussed above, the emphasis of this book is on the inferential concepts used to interpret samples, rather than a detailed study of the ways samples are generated, but it is still useful to bear in mind the underlying complexity of the random sampling process.

Example 1.5 In Example 1.2 we discussed a study in which individuals presenting at a hospital with a heart attack are observed for a one month period to determine whether they survive over this period. This is an example of a prospective sample, because individuals are identified at the time of presenting to the hospital with a heart attack, and then they are followed forward in time to assess whether they survived. A retrospective sample for the same context could be obtained by looking up the hospital records to find historical cases of heart attack patients and their corresponding survival status after one month. Thus, in contrast to the prospective sample, the retrospective sample would involve looking back in time to obtain the sample. In both cases the goal would be to assess the risk of death which, as discussed in Example 1.2, is the probability of death over the specific time frame of interest. Another important use of probability in biostatistics is to measure **prevalence**, which is undertaken using cross-sectional sampling. The prevalence of a particular attribute in the population is a measure of the extent of that attribute, and is defined simply as the proportion of the population that has that attribute. Prevalence can therefore be interpreted as a probability, in that it will correspond with the relative frequency in a large sample from the population. Commonly we use prevalence to measure the extent of a particular disease, although in principle it can also be used to measure the extent of any other attribute. The prevalence of disease is assessed using a **prevalence sample**, also sometimes called a survey, which is a sample where each individual is assessed for their current disease status. Such samples are cross-sectional, in the sense that information is obtained about current disease status, but no information about previous or future experiences is obtained. Thus, a cross-sectional prevalence sample can be thought of as a snapshot of the current extent of the disease within the population. The **sample prevalence** is then simply the proportion of the sample that has the disease of interest. In subsequent examples we will use the sample prevalence as a tool for making inferences about the population prevalence.

1.8   Sampling bias

In the previous section we discussed random samples in which all individuals in the population have the same probability of being included in the sample. When this is the case then the random sample can be considered representative of the population. Sometimes, however, this may not be the case. That is, sometimes we may have a sample in which some individuals from the population were more likely to be included than others. In this case the sample is not representative of the population and the rationale for using the sample to make inferences about the population is no longer valid. We refer to such a situation as **sampling bias**.

If it is known exactly how individuals differ with respect to their probability of being included in the sample, then it is possible to incorporate this knowledge into the statistical inference process. This may allow us to validly account for the sampling bias in our inferences about the population. However, if it is not known exactly how the individuals differ with respect to their inclusion probabilities then the lack of representativeness of the sample cannot be accounted for. This may lead to invalid, or biased, inferences about the population. When sampling bias exists in biostatistical applications it is not common to know exactly how individuals differ with respect to their probability of being included in the sample, so it is always best to avoid sampling bias in the first place.

As an illustration of sampling bias, suppose that we were interested in assessing the prevalence of HIV infection in a particular population, and we took our prevalence sample from among those individuals who have a screening test at a sexually transmitted disease (STD) clinic in that population. Then this would be an unrepresentative sample because not all people in the population would have the same chance of being included in the sample. In particular, those individuals with an STD would have a greater chance of being sampled, and this would lead to our sample having an over-representation of individuals with HIV infection. In this context, any inferences arising from our sample would relate to the population of individuals that present to the STD clinic, not the general population that we are interested in. That is, our inferences would be valid for the wrong population and invalid for the right population.

While sampling bias is a very important issue in biostatistics, particularly in epidemiological studies, in this book we will generally focus on how to make inferences about populations based on samples that are representative of the population. Nonetheless, it is important to remember that statistical inference techniques may lead to invalid conclusions if the sample is systematically biased in some way.

1.9 Sampling variation

Although we may be satisfied that our sampling process was truly random, so that sampling bias is not present, our sample will still be subject to random variation in the sense that if we took two different samples from the same population they would not give exactly the same results. For example, we may be satisfied that the sample prevalence is not likely to be systematically higher or lower than the population prevalence, but in different samples the sample prevalence would be expected to vary in a random fashion. If this random variation is "large" then we would place less trust in the inferences from our sample than if the random variation was "small". The random variation exhibited by our sample is referred to as **sampling variation**. A key element of statistical inference is the quantification of sampling variability, so that we have some indication of how much we trust the sample as a basis for making inferences about the population.

The following example based on cross-sectional prevalence sampling illustrates the effect of sampling variation, and it introduces us to the idea of describing the sampling variation using probability. Our approach will be to use an appropriate probability distribution as a model for the random variation inherent in our sampling process. This then leads to a way of measuring the magnitude of sampling variation using the variability exhibited by this probability distribution. While the following example provides us with an introduction to the use of probability to model sampling variation, this modelling process is at the heart of statistical inference and will be taken up in more generality in the next chapter.

Example 1.6 As an illustration of sampling variability, consider the effect of sample size on a prevalence sample. If we calculated the sample prevalence using a sample of 100 individuals, we would naturally trust it less than if it had been based on a sample of 1000 individuals. In other words, we would expect the prevalence in a sample of 100 individuals to vary less from sample to sample than the prevalence in a sample of 1000 individuals. To see this, consider the results of 10 different studies, each of which involved taking a random sample of 100 individuals and observing their infection status. Although we would not know this in practice, suppose that the prevalence in the population is 15%. Figure 1.3 displays a plot of the 10 sample prevalences. The first point to notice is that the 10 sample prevalences are bunched around the true population prevalence, some higher and some lower. This is indicative of a representative or unbiased sampling scheme. Importantly, however, each individual study yields a sample prevalence that differs from the population prevalence of 15%, and the range of estimates in this series of 10 studies is 9.0% to 20.0%. It is the extent of this variation around the true population prevalence that reflects the sampling variation, and clearly we would trust our sample prevalence more if this sampling variation were lower. Next consider a similar series of 10 prevalence studies, with the exception that each includes 1000 individuals in the sample instead of 100. These 10 samples are also plotted in Figure 1.3. Again the sample prevalence values are bunched around the population prevalence of 15%, and again each individual sample prevalence value differs from the population value. This time, however, the variation about the population prevalence is lower than it was in the smaller samples, and ranges from 13.5% to 16.7% across the samples. This illustrates that the larger prevalence samples tend to have less sampling variation, or more accuracy, than the smaller samples.

One part of the statistical inference process is to summarise our trust in the sample by taking into account the magnitude and nature of this sampling variability. In order to summarise the variability inherent in our sample, we first use a model based on a probability distribution to describe the variability. The specific probability distribution we use will depend on the context and we will discuss this in some detail in subsequent chapters. For our prevalence sample in this example, the binomial distribution provides a natural model for the way the sampling has been carried out. Let n be the sample size in our prevalence study, and let T be the number of individuals who are found to have the disease in our sample. Then the sample prevalence is $P = T/n$. Under our study design n is a fixed number, or a constant, since we had planned to sample a certain fixed number of individuals from the population. Thus n is not subject to any random variation. T on the other hand will vary randomly from sample to sample, and is therefore a random variable. Under our binomial sampling scheme, the nature of this random variation in T is governed by the binomial distribution, $\mathrm{Bin}(n, \theta)$, where θ is the true population prevalence. In particular,

$$\Pr(T = t) = \frac{n!}{(n-t)!t!} \theta^t (1-\theta)^{n-t} \qquad t = 0, 1, \ldots, n.$$

As we noted in Example 1.3, the binomial model is appropriate under the assumption that the infection statuses of different individuals are independent. Given the repeated sampling interpretation of probability, the binomial probability distribution specifies how we expect the number of infected individuals to vary in repeated samples of size n. We can therefore use this probability distribution to summarise our level of trust in the sample prevalence as an indication of the population prevalence. In particular, since we will have more trust in our sample if it leads to less variation from sample to sample, the variance associated with the sample prevalence is a natural way to summarise the sampling variation. Using our knowledge of the binomial distribution summarised in Appendix 1, as well as the properties of variances discussed in Section 1.4,

$$\mathrm{Var}(P) = \mathrm{Var}\left(\frac{T}{n}\right) = \frac{n\theta(1-\theta)}{n^2} = \frac{\theta(1-\theta)}{n}.$$

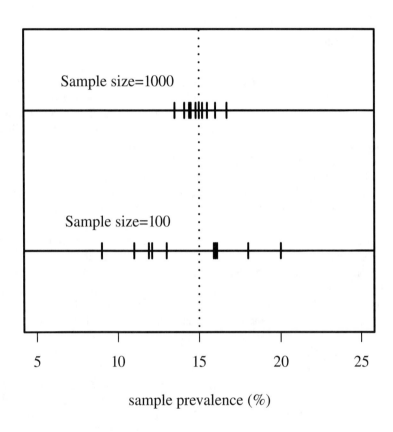

FIGURE 1.3
Sample prevalence in 10 prevalence samples of size 100, and 10 prevalence samples of size 1000

From this it can be seen that the variance of the sample prevalence is inversely related to the sample size n. That is, the sample prevalence will be less variable in studies with larger sample sizes. This explains the behaviour we saw in Figure 1.3 above. In Chapter 2 we will discuss more elaborate ways to summarise the sampling variability, which will lead us to one of the most important inferential tools, the confidence interval.

1.10   Large samples

Building on Example 1.6, in the coming chapters we will discuss at some length the use of probability to model sampling variation exhibited by random variables in our sample. One of the central themes will be that certain random variables can be used to estimate important attributes of our population, and hence to produce inferences about our population. This process, which we will call estimation, is facilitated by using the probability distribution of these random variables to describe their behaviour. As was illustrated in Example 1.6, this allows us to quantify the sampling variability and summarise the level of trust that we place in our inferences.

The particular probability model that we use is key to our understanding of the nature of the sampling variability. In principle, different probability models will lead to different descriptions of the sampling variability, and hence potentially lead to different inferences. However, in large samples there is an important result from probability theory that says our sampling variability can be described using the normal distribution, regardless of the underlying probability model. This leads to a central unifying theme in our subsequent discussions, which is that the probability distributions of random variables used to estimate population characteristics can be approximated by the normal distribution in large samples. This simplifies our inference process by yielding an approximate approach that can be applied in many situations where the sample is large but where the natural probability distribution is not the normal distribution. We will see that this provides a unified approach to statistical inference across a very wide range of otherwise unrelated contexts. The details of these large sample simplifications will be introduced in subsequent chapters. However, before we can do this, we need to state some important probabilistic concepts and properties that will form the basis of the normal approximations that hold in large samples.

In the context of statistical inference based on a random sample, we have said that we will be interested in certain random variables whose value is determined by the sample. The large sample probabilistic behaviour of such random variables will be studied by considering the way they behave as the sample size n increases. This will require us to think about a sequence of random variables, indexed by the sample size n. A natural example of such a sequence is the sample mean indexed by n,

$$\overline{X}_n = \frac{1}{n}\sum_{i=1}^{n} X_i.$$

In this case, the sequence of random variables $\overline{X}_1, \overline{X}_2, \ldots, \overline{X}_n, \ldots$ represents the sample means from samples of increasing sample size. The large sample behaviour of the sample mean is therefore specified by the limiting behaviour of this sequence as $n \to \infty$. Consideration of the "limit" of a sequence of random variables introduces us to the concept of **convergence of random variables**, which we now discuss in more detail.

In mathematics, the notion of convergence of a non-random sequence $x_1, x_2, \ldots$ to a limit c, written as

$$x_n \to c \qquad \text{or} \qquad \lim_{n \to \infty} x_n = c,$$

represents the idea that the sequence of values x_n approaches a particular constant value c as $n \to \infty$. In that context, there is an unambiguous mathematical definition of what it means for the non-random sequence to converge to c. For a sequence of random variables, however, the notion of convergence can mean many things, so there is no single way to define convergence of the sequence. Indeed, it turns out that there are many types of convergence used in probability theory, usually called **modes of convergence**, but two in particular will suffice for our purposes.

The first mode of convergence is called **convergence in distribution**. This type of convergence specifies that the probability distribution of X_n converges to the probability distribution of some random variable X as $n \to \infty$, and it is written as

$$X_n \xrightarrow{d} X.$$

More precisely, convergence in distribution is defined via the cumulative distributions functions of X_n and X, which we will denote by $F_n(x)$ and $F(x)$, respectively. Using the cumulative distribution functions, convergence in distribution is defined as

$$\lim_{n \to \infty} F_n(x) = F(x) \qquad \text{for all } x \in (-\infty, \infty).$$

The most important example of convergence in distribution is the **Central Limit Theorem**. Consider an independent random sample $X_1, \ldots, X_n$, in which each X_i has the same distribution with $E(X_i) = \mu$ and $Var(X_i) = \sigma^2$. Then, regardless of the actual distribution of X_i, the Central Limit Theorem says that the standardised version of the sample mean

$$Z_n = \frac{\overline{X}_n - \mu}{\sigma / \sqrt{n}}$$

converges in distribution to a standard normal random variable

$$Z_n \xrightarrow{d} N(0, 1).$$

In the context of statistical inference, an important use of convergence in distribution is that it provides us with an approximate distribution when the sample size n is sufficiently large. Thus, for example, the Central Limit Theorem allows us to specify the approximate distribution of the sample mean in large samples, which is written as

$$\overline{X}_n \stackrel{d}{\approx} N\left(\mu, \frac{\sigma^2}{n}\right) \qquad \text{for large } n$$

where the notation $\stackrel{d}{\approx}$ means "is approximately distributed as". We will see that many of the techniques discussed in this book are large sample methods that can be justified by the Central Limit Theorem or one of its variants.

The second mode of convergence is called **convergence in probability**. This type of convergence, which is written as

$$X_n \stackrel{p}{\to} X,$$

specifies that the probability of X_n being close to X converges to 1 as $n \to \infty$, no matter how strictly we define "close". More precisely, convergence in probability is defined as

$$\Pr\left(|X_n - X| < \varepsilon\right) \longrightarrow 1 \qquad \text{as } n \longrightarrow \infty$$

for any value $\varepsilon > 0$, no matter how small.

An important special case of convergence in probability is when the random variable X is a constant, also called a **degenerate random variable**, in which case $\Pr(X = c) = 1$ for some constant c. In this case the sequence of random variables converges in probability to a constant

$$X_n \stackrel{p}{\longrightarrow} c.$$

An important example of convergence in probability to a constant is the **Law of Large Numbers**. For the independent random sample used to state the Central Limit Theorem above, the Law of Large Numbers says that the sample mean converges in probability to μ, written as

$$\overline{X}_n \stackrel{p}{\longrightarrow} \mu.$$

The notion of convergence in probability to a constant will be important in subsequent chapters for describing the large sample behaviour of random variables that are used to estimate population characteristics on the basis of a random sample. For example, the Law of Large Numbers states that the sample mean $\overline{X}_n$ will have a tendency to be close to the population mean μ in large samples, which is clearly a desirable estimation property. This type of property also extends to other sample analogues of population quantities. For example, it will be seen in Chapter 2 that the sample variance

$$S_n^2 = \frac{1}{n}\sum_{i=1}^{n}\left(X_i - \overline{X}_n\right)^2$$

will have a tendency to be close to the population variance σ^2 in large samples.

It is natural to ask whether convergence in distribution and convergence in probability are distinct types of convergence, that is, whether it is possible to have one without the other. In fact, convergence in distribution can be thought of as a weaker

Probability and random samples   29

form of convergence than convergence in probability, in the sense that the latter implies the former. In other words, it can be proved that $X_n \xrightarrow{P} X$ implies $X_n \xrightarrow{d} X$, but the reverse is not necessarily true. As alluded to earlier, other modes of convergence of random variables also exist, including modes that are stronger than convergence in probability, but we will not need to discuss these in this book.

Example 1.7 In previous examples we considered the random variable $P = T/n$, which is the sample prevalence of an infection in a random sample of n individuals, T of which are observed to have the infection present. In Example 1.6 we specified a binomial distribution for T, which is equivalent to saying that P has a probability distribution specified by the probability function

$$f_P(p) = \Pr(P = p) = \frac{n!}{(n-pn)!(pn)!} \theta^{pn}(1-\theta)^{n-pn} \qquad p = 0, \frac{1}{n}, \frac{2}{n}, \dots, 1.$$

The random variable P is the mean of n binary variables taking the values 0 or 1, each indicating whether the infection is absent or present, respectively, for the n individuals in the random sample. We can therefore use the Central Limit Theorem to approximate the distribution of P. This leads to the approximate distribution

$$P \stackrel{d}{\approx} N\left(\theta, \frac{\theta(1-\theta)}{n}\right) \qquad \text{for large } n.$$

This large sample approximation follows from the fact that the standardised version of P converges in distribution to a standard normal random variable as the sample size increases, that is

$$\frac{P - \theta}{\sqrt{\theta(1-\theta)/n}} \xrightarrow{d} N(0,1).$$

The approximate normal distribution for P is an approximation to the "exact" distribution specified by the probability function $f_P(p)$. The importance of this large sample approximate distribution is that it is much simpler to make use of for inferential purposes, and the same approach can be used in many other inferential contexts. We will discuss this at some length in Chapter 2, along with the importance of various other large sample properties. For example, in Chapter 2 we will also focus on the significance of the fact that the Law of Large Numbers implies that $P \xrightarrow{P} \theta$, meaning that the sample prevalence will have a tendency to be close to the population prevalence in large samples.

To see the normal approximation in practice, suppose we continued the series of studies that we summarised in Figure 1.3. Suppose, instead of conducting just 10 studies each involving prevalence samples of size $n = 1000$, we now conducted 10,000 studies each with a sample size $n = 1000$. The observed sample prevalence from each of these studies is an observation from the binomial model for the sampling variability P, as specified by the probability function $f_P(p)$. Figure 1.4 shows a histogram of how the observed prevalence values vary from study to study. Also shown is the expected number of studies within each range of sample prevalence

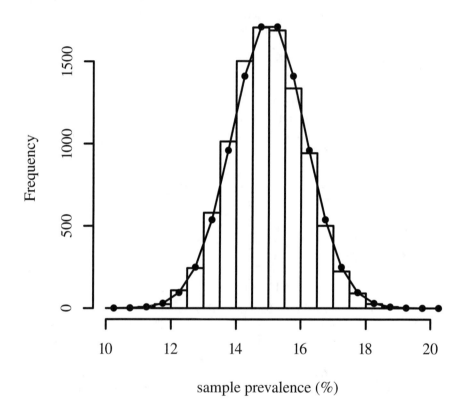

FIGURE 1.4
Histogram of observed sample prevalence in 10,000 samples, and the number expected using the large sample normal approximation

values, according to the normal approximation. It can be seen that the normal approximation, arising from the Central Limit Theorem, does indeed provide a good approximation for the distribution of the sample prevalence. As alluded to earlier, large sample normal approximations such as this will form the basis of many of the statistical inference methods that we discuss in subsequent chapters.

Exercises

1. In this exercise we will carry out probability calculations for the normal distribution. You will need a way of evaluating the standard normal cumulative distribution function $\Phi(z)$. One way to do this is using the R computing environment described in Appendix 2, using the command pnorm(z).

   (a) For a standard normal random variable $Z \overset{d}{=} N(0,1)$, calculate the probabilities $\Pr(Z \leq -2)$ and $\Pr(Z > 1)$. Hence give the probability $\Pr(-2 < Z \leq 1)$.

   (b) Plot the function $\Phi(z)$ and mark areas corresponding to each of the three probabilities from part (a).

   (c) Repeat part (a) for the $N(1,5)$ and $N(-1,5)$ distributions, after first converting the required probability statements into statements about the standard normal distribution.

   (d) For $Y \overset{d}{=} N(5,2.5)$ calculate the probability $\Pr(4.5 \leq Y \leq 5.5)$. As in part (c), first convert this probability statement into a statement about the standard normal distribution.

   (e) Repeat part (d) for $Y \overset{d}{=} N(5,5)$.

   (f) With the aid of a graph, explain why your answer to part (d) is greater than your answer to part (e).

2. In this exercise we will carry out probability calculations for the binomial and Poisson distributions. These calculations can be carried out directly using the probability functions provided in Appendix 1, or using the dbinom and dpois functions in R.

   (a) For $Y \overset{d}{=} Bin(10,0.5)$ calculate the probability $\Pr(Y = 5)$. Comment on the result in relation to Exercise 1(d).

   (b) For $Y \overset{d}{=} Pois(5)$ calculate the probability $\Pr(Y = 5)$. Comment on the result in relation to Exercise 1(e).

   (c) Show that if a binomial distribution and a Poisson distribution have the same mean, then the Poisson distribution has greater variance.

   (d) Plot the probability functions of the $Bin(10,0.5)$ and $Pois(5)$ distributions and comment on the results in relation to part (c).

3. In Table 1.2 we calculated the probability distribution of the random variable T, the number infected in a sample of size two, based on the first assignment of event probabilities from Table 1.1.

   (a) Repeat the probability distribution calculations in Table 1.2 using the second assignment of probabilities from Table 1.1.

   (b) Based on the probability distribution from part (a), calculate the mean and the variance of T.

   (c) Show that T has a $\mathrm{Bin}(2,0.55)$ distribution, by evaluating the probability function of this distribution.

   (d) Use the properties of the binomial distribution to state the mean and variance of T directly, and confirm that these are consistent with the calculations in part (b).

4. Consider Example 1.4, in which we studied T from Exercise 3 above, as well as T_1 and T_2, the infection statuses of the first and second individuals in the sample, respectively. In Example 1.4 we used the first probability assignment from Table 1.1. In this exercise we will use the second probability assignment from Table 1.1.

   (a) Write down $\Pr(\mathscr{E}_0) = \Pr(T = 1)$, $\Pr(\mathscr{E}_1) = \Pr(T_1 = 1)$ and $\Pr(\mathscr{E}_2) = \Pr(T_2 = 1)$.

   (b) Show that $\mathscr{E}_1$ and $\mathscr{E}_2$ are independent events.

   (c) Show that $\mathscr{E}_1$ and $\mathscr{E}_0$ are not independent events.

   (d) Evaluate the joint probability function $f_{T_1,T_2}(t_1,t_2)$ for the four possible combinations of $t_1 = 0,1$ and $t_2 = 0,1$. Hence show that T_1 and T_2 are independent random variables.

5. In this exercise you will need a way to simulate normally distributed observations. One way to do this is using the rnorm function in R, which is described in Appendix 2.

   (a) Simulate a random sample of size $n = 20$ from the standard normal distribution and calculate the sample mean. If you are using R you can do this with the single command mean(rnorm(20)).

   (b) Repeat your simulation from part (a) until you have 10 simulated sample means. Mark your simulated sample means on a graph analogous to Figure 1.3.

   (c) Repeat part (b) for $n = 100$, $n = 1000$ and $n = 10,000$. For each collection of 10 simulations, mark your simulations on the graph from part (b), similarly to Figure 1.3.

   (d) What does your graph say about sampling variability? Explain your observation with reference to the Law of Large Numbers.

(e) Write down a theoretical expression for $\mathrm{Var}(\overline{Z}_n)$, where $\overline{Z}_n$ is the sample mean from a random sample of n standard normal random variables. Explain how this theoretical expression concords with your simulation results.

6. In this exercise we consider disease incidence studies. Whereas prevalence studies allow assessment of the extent of *existing* disease, incidence studies assess the rate of occurrence of *new* cases of disease. Rather than the cross-sectional sampling scheme used in prevalence samples, the sampling scheme in an incidence study is generally prospective. That is, a cohort of individuals is followed over time, and new cases of disease are recorded. The **incidence rate** is the rate of occurrence of new cases of disease per unit of time per individual.

We will use the following notation. Let n be the total number of individuals and let X be the number of individuals who experience onset of the disease during the observation period, also called the follow-up period. Let F_i be the number of years that individual i is followed for, with $F = \sum_i F_i$ being the aggregate number of years that the cohort is followed for. The n individuals are therefore followed for an average of $A = F/n$ years, and we say that the cohort has been followed for F person-years. The rate of occurrence of new cases of disease per year of follow-up will be labelled λ, and we will call this the population incidence rate. Thus, the expected number of new disease events is $\mathrm{E}(X) = \lambda F$. This exercise will make use of the simulation function inc.sim for the R computing environment, as described in Appendix 2.

(a) Suppose that X has a Poisson distribution. Write down the probability function for X.

(b) We will call $R = X/F$ the sample incidence rate. Using part (a), write down the probability function of R.

(c) Using properties of the Poisson distribution, and properties of expectations and variances, write down $\mathrm{E}(R)$ and $\mathrm{Var}(R)$.

(d) Explain why the sample incidence rate R is a sensible estimate of the population incidence rate λ. Explain why the sampling variability of R will be smaller when the total follow-up F is larger.

(e) The Poisson distribution can be approximated by the normal distribution when its mean is large. Write down a normal approximation to the probability distribution of R, after first writing down a normal approximation to the distribution of X.

(f) Use the simulation function inc.sim described in Appendix 2 to carry out 10,000 simulations of R based on Poisson sampling, assuming that the population incidence rate is 15 events per 1000 years of follow-up, and we follow 350 individuals for an average of 5 years. Using these simulations, verify that the probability distribution of R is approximately normal using a histogram.

7. In Section 1.6 we wrote down the bivariate normal joint probability density function, $f_{X,Y}(x,y) = f_{\mathbf{X}}(\mathbf{x})$, associated with bivariate normal random variables X and Y.

   (a) By expanding the term $(\mathbf{x} - \boldsymbol{\mu})^T \Sigma^{-1}(\mathbf{x} - \boldsymbol{\mu})$ that appears in the joint density function, express the joint density function in terms of x and y. You will need to review the definition of a matrix inverse for a 2×2 matrix.

   (b) Suppose now that X and Y are two independent normal random variables. Write down the joint probability density function and the joint cumulative distribution function of X and Y. Use the notation $\Phi(z)$ for the standard normal cumulative distribution function.

   (c) By simplifying the function from part (a), write down $f_{X,Y}(x,y)$ when $\rho = 0$. Hence, using part (b), show that when $\rho = 0$ then X and Y are independent. This is a special property of the bivariate normal distribution, and in general it is not true that zero correlation implies independence.

2

Estimation concepts

In this chapter we build on our previous discussion of sampling from a population to obtain information about that population. We discuss in more detail the concept of a statistical model for a random sample, which is a probability distribution that depends on characteristics of the population and the way in which we took our sample from the population. The focus of the chapter is estimation of unknown quantities associated with this probability distribution, called parameters, which represent characteristics of interest within the population. We limit our discussion in this chapter to properties of given estimation procedures and criteria for assessing their usefulness. In subsequent chapters we will broaden this to discuss general methods for deriving estimation procedures, and for drawing inferences about the unknown parameters. The concepts are briefly illustrated using our disease prevalence example from Chapter 1, and are then exemplified in greater detail using an extended example on modelling a continuous risk factor.

2.1 Statistical models

We have seen that statistical inference involves an observed sample, usually referred to as the data, which is assumed to have arisen through a process of random sampling from a population of interest. The population is considered to be unobservable in its entirety, for example because it is too large, and the primary concern is to use the observed sample to gain information about the unobservable population. In Chapter 1 we discussed a number of ways in which samples are commonly obtained in biostatistical applications. We also discussed the broader interpretation of a random sample that is required when our data did not arise by literally sampling individuals at random from a population.

With those basic concepts in hand, the next step is to understand how we use the observed data to draw inferences about the unobservable population. Our inference process begins with a **statistical model** which describes the potential outcomes of our random sampling process. Formally, a statistical model involves viewing the sample y as being the observed value of a random variable Y. Less formally, this means that the data can be thought of as arising from a process that could give rise to a wide range of possible values, whose distribution can be characterised using probabilities. The statistical model specifies the probability distribution that the random variable

Y is assumed to follow, which will be a continuous probability density function for a continuous outcome, or a discrete probability function for a discrete outcome. We will denote both of these by $f_Y(y)$, which specifies the distribution of the sample.

The probability distribution $f_Y(y)$, which provides the model for our data, depends on both the characteristics of the population that we are interested in, as well as the way in which we took our sample from the population. Importantly, because we lack complete knowledge of the population, the distribution of Y is not completely known. Statistical inference is concerned with using y to make inferences about the unknown aspects of $f_Y(y)$, and hence about the population of interest.

The observed sample y will usually be a composite entity, not a single observation. Typically it will be a vector of observations, $y = (y_1, \ldots, y_n)$, which is the observed value of a vector of random variables $Y = (Y_1, \ldots, Y_n)$. Often in biostatistics these observations are from n different individuals, in which case it is usually assumed that $Y_1, \ldots, Y_n$ are independent random variables. This simplifies our model, because it means that $f_Y(y)$ depends only on the distributions associated with each individual, $f_i(y_i)$. In particular, it means the joint probability distribution $f_Y(y)$ will take the simplified form

$$f_Y(y) = f_1(y_1)f_2(y_2)\ldots f_n(y_n) = \prod_{i=1}^{n} f_i(y_i).$$

Most of the examples that we discuss in this book will be for situations where the observations come from independent random variables. When this assumption is not reasonable, such as when there are multiple observations on each individual, a more complex probability model will be needed that incorporates dependencies between the observations in our sample. Although a detailed study of such models goes beyond the scope of this book, many of the general inference methods that we will discuss continue to be applicable for more complex models and so they provide a precursor to the study of more advance methods.

Before illustrating the concept of a statistical model using a concrete example, we highlight a very important class of models that will primarily occupy us in this book.

2.2   Parametric models

A large part of statistical inference is concerned with statistical models that assume the distribution of our sample Y takes a particular form that is assumed known except for a small number of fixed unknown constants, called **parameters**. Once these parameters are specified the full distribution of the sample is specified. This is referred to as a **parametric model**. Using parametric models, statistical inference reduces to estimating and testing hypotheses about the unknown parameters, which usually represent important unknown characteristics of the population that the sample was taken from. To denote the dependence of our model on the parameters, we use the notation $f_Y(y;\theta)$, where θ may be a single parameter or a vector of parameters $\theta = (\theta_1,\ldots,\theta_p)$. The set of all possible values for the parameter θ is called the **parameter space**. The set of all possible values for the observed sample y is called the sample space, a term that we introduced in the context of probability in Chapter 1.

For concreteness and ease of presentation, this chapter will assume that there is just a single parameter, unless otherwise stated. This means that θ is a one-dimensional quantity. However, all of the concepts we discuss in this chapter also have relevance when θ is a vector. We will briefly illustrate this in the extended example at the end of this chapter, and then in Chapter 4 we will fully generalise our discussion to a multiple parameter context.

Example 2.1 Consider the prevalence sample that we discussed in the examples from Chapter 1. In this case there was a single parameter θ, the unknown prevalence of the disease in the population, and the parameter space is the interval $[0,1]$. The parameter θ can be interpreted as the prevalence that we would observe if we were able to study an infinitely large sample of individuals. The sample consists of n observations $y = (y_1,\ldots,y_n)$ where $y_i = 1$ if individual i has the disease, and $y_i = 0$ if individual i does not have the disease. Assuming that our random sample has been taken such that all individuals in the population have the same probability of being sampled, then the probability function for the observation from individual i is

$$f_i(y_i;\theta) = \Pr(Y_i = y_i) = \theta^{y_i}(1-\theta)^{1-y_i} \qquad y_i = 0,1.$$

This leads to the following model for the complete sample

$$f_Y(y;\theta) = \Pr(Y = y) = \prod_{i=1}^{n} \theta^{y_i}(1-\theta)^{1-y_i}.$$

It is important to remember that this model is based on the assumption that all individuals have equal probability of being sampled, and we would need to use a different model if this was not true. Most of the examples in this book will be based on this assumption, but in Section 1.8 we discussed some of the consequences of taking our sample in other ways. Notice also that the above model does not have the same form as the distribution we used to model the prevalence sample in Chapter 1. There we condensed the sample down to a single random variable $T = \sum_{i=1}^{n} Y_i$ with observed value $t = \sum_{i=1}^{n} y_i$ representing the total number of individuals in the sample that have the disease. We then modelled this single random variable using the binomial probability model

$$f_T(t;\theta) = \Pr(T = t) = \frac{n!}{(n-t)!t!}\theta^t(1-\theta)^{n-t}.$$

These two approaches turn out to be equivalent, and the condensing of our sample from a vector down to a sum introduces us to the idea of data reduction, which takes a central place in statistical inference and will be discussed in the next section.

2.3 Statistics and data reduction

Any function of our sample that does not depend on θ, say $T(Y)$, is referred to as a **statistic**, and is itself a random variable. By this we mean any quantity or quantities that can be calculated from Y. The observed value of the random variable, $t = T(y)$, is referred to as the observed sample value of the statistic. One example of a statistic is the sum of the individual observations $T(Y) = \sum_{i=1}^{n} Y_i$, while another example is the sum of the squares of the observations $T(Y) = \sum_{i=1}^{n} Y_i^2$. Because a statistic is a function of the sample, the distribution of the sample determines the distribution of the statistic, and this distribution will depend on the parameter θ. Thus, it will be possible, and in some cases more convenient, to base our inference about θ on the distribution of the statistic, $f_T(t; \theta)$, rather than the distribution of the entire sample, $f_Y(y; \theta)$. This is what we did in Example 2.1 and Chapter 1 by using the binomial model for the sum of the individual observations. Note that a statistic can potentially be a vector, for example $T(Y) = (\sum_{i=1}^{n} Y_i, \sum_{i=1}^{n} Y_i^2)$.

The use of a statistic as the basis of our inference corresponds to data reduction in the sense that it is not necessary to know the complete sample to carry out our inferences. This leads to a natural question: to what extent has important information been lost by reducing our sample down to a statistic? In Chapter 3 we will study this question in more detail and discuss how we can know whether a statistic is "sufficient" for conveying all the available information in the sample. However, for now we assume that nothing important has been lost by reducing our sample down to a statistic, and focus on the use of sample statistics as the basis for estimating the unknown parameters of our model.

2.4 Estimators and estimates

The fundamental problem in statistical estimation is to choose a value for the parameter θ that is close to the true unknown value. The value that we choose will be based on the observed sample y and is called an **estimate** for θ. For any given approach to calculating an estimate of θ, our goal is to study the statistical properties of the approach, for example its behaviour on average. By describing the statistical properties of the estimation procedure, we are able to assess whether the procedure is useful, for example, whether it is likely to produce an estimate that is close to the true parameter value. To this end, we consider an estimate to be the observed value of a particular statistic, which we call an **estimator**. The probability distribution of the estimator, called the **sampling distribution**, gives us information on how the estimator behaves in repeated samples from the same population. This allows us to assess whether the estimator is useful for producing an estimate of θ. For example, it would make sense to require, at a minimum, that the mean of the distribution of our estimator is close to the true value of θ, so that on average over a large number of studies, we know that our estimate will be close to θ.

In order to consider more clearly the distinction between an estimator and an estimate, recall that the observed sample y is regarded as the observed value of a random variable Y. The estimate of θ, which we will write as $\hat{\theta}$, is a function of the observed sample, so that $\hat{\theta} = \Theta(y)$, for some function Θ. On the other hand, the estimator, which we will write as $\hat{\Theta}$, is a function of the random variable Y, so that $\hat{\Theta} = \Theta(Y)$. Thus, the estimator is a statistic, and the estimate is the observed value of this statistic, or the sample value of the statistic. The distribution of $\hat{\Theta}$, the sampling distribution, is the distribution that we are interested in for describing the properties of the estimator.

As a specific example of this notation for distinguishing between parameters, estimates and estimators, consider a population mean μ, which might be estimated by the sample mean $\bar{y}$. Then μ is the parameter and $\bar{y}$ is the estimate. Furthermore, the estimate $\bar{y}$ is considered to be the observed value of a random variable $\bar{Y}$, which is the estimator. This leads to the notational correspondence

$$\theta = \mu \qquad \hat{\theta} = \bar{y} \qquad \hat{\Theta} = \bar{Y}.$$

We will return to this estimation context in greater detail in the extended example. For now, however, we will look at an example of estimates and estimators in our familiar binomial prevalence sampling problem, before going on to discuss in detail the types of properties that useful estimators should possess.

Example 2.2 Using the notation of our prevalence example, the observed sample reduces to the observed number of individuals y who have the disease, and this is modelled as the observed value of a random variable Y that has a $\text{Bin}(n, \theta)$ distribution. For a particular sample, the estimate of θ is

$$\hat{\theta} = p = \frac{y}{n}.$$

Thus, in a particular sample, say with 121 diseased individuals out of 1000, the estimate takes on a specific value, say 0.121. This value is the observed value of a random variable, the estimator of θ, which is

$$\hat{\Theta} = P = \frac{Y}{n}.$$

In the hypothetical repeated sampling that underlies the statistical model, this random variable has a probability distribution, or sampling distribution, that we specified in Chapter 1.

2.5 Properties of estimators

The first quantity of interest associated with the distribution of the estimator $\hat{\Theta}$ is its mean, or expectation, $E(\hat{\Theta})$. Ideally, this should be equal to the true parameter value θ, or at least be quite close to this value. When $E(\hat{\Theta}) = \theta$ we say that $\hat{\Theta}$ is an **unbiased estimator** of θ. If an estimator is unbiased then it has no systematic tendency to under- or over-estimate the unknown parameter value. If it is not unbiased then we refer to it as a **biased estimator**. The quantity

$$\text{Bias}(\hat{\Theta}) = E(\hat{\Theta}) - \theta$$

is referred to as the **bias** of the estimator. Thus, unbiased estimators have a bias of zero. While unbiasedness is clearly a desirable property of estimators, in practice we often tolerate estimators that have a small bias, particularly if they have other desirable properties.

The property of unbiasedness is concerned with the average value of the estimator. A second property of interest is the variability of the estimator, which can be quantified by its variance. In fact, for reasons that will become apparent when we talk about confidence intervals later in the chapter, we often focus on the square root of an estimator's variance, called the **standard error**

$$\text{SE}(\hat{\Theta}) = \sqrt{\text{Var}(\hat{\Theta})}.$$

A desirable property of an estimator is that it has a "small" standard error, as this indicates that the estimator does not vary very much. In particular, if a small standard error is combined with unbiasedness then the estimator will tend to take values that are close to θ. If we had to make a choice between two competing unbiased estimators in order to calculate an estimate of θ, then we would choose the one with the smallest variance, or equivalently the smallest standard error. This suggests a numerical way of comparing different unbiased estimators. Given two different unbiased estimators of θ, $\hat{\Theta}_1$ and $\hat{\Theta}_2$, the **efficiency** of $\hat{\Theta}_1$ relative to $\hat{\Theta}_2$ is

$$\text{Eff}(\hat{\Theta}_1, \hat{\Theta}_2) = \frac{\text{Var}(\hat{\Theta}_2)}{\text{Var}(\hat{\Theta}_1)}.$$

Thus, if $\text{Eff}(\hat{\Theta}_1, \hat{\Theta}_2) > 1$ then $\hat{\Theta}_1$ would be preferred to $\hat{\Theta}_2$.

An important result in theoretical statistics tells us that there is a limit to how well an unbiased estimator can perform in terms of variability. For any unbiased estimator $\hat{\Theta}$,

$$\text{Var}(\hat{\Theta}) \geq I(\theta)^{-1} = -E\left[\frac{d^2}{d\theta^2}\log f_Y(Y;\theta)\right]^{-1}.$$

This is called the **minimum variance bound** (or the **Cramér-Rao bound**) and it gives a lower limit for the variance of an unbiased estimator. In words, it states that the variance of an unbiased estimator is no smaller than the negative of the inverse of the expectation of the second derivative of the log of the probability (density) function of the sample. Any unbiased estimator with a variance that attains this bound is the least variable of all unbiased estimators, and is said to be **efficient**.

As noted above, we do not always restrict ourselves to unbiased estimators. However, if we wish to compare estimators that may be biased, then we need to take into account both the magnitude of the bias, as well as the magnitude of the variability. A simultaneous measure of both the bias and variability of an estimator is provided by the **mean squared error**

$$\text{MSE}(\hat{\Theta}) = \text{E}\left[(\hat{\Theta} - \theta)^2\right] = \text{Bias}(\hat{\Theta})^2 + \text{Var}(\hat{\Theta}).$$

This leads to an alternative measure of efficiency for comparing estimators

$$\text{Eff}(\hat{\Theta}_1, \hat{\Theta}_2) = \frac{\text{MSE}(\hat{\Theta}_2)}{\text{MSE}(\hat{\Theta}_1)}.$$

If either of the estimators is biased then this measure of efficiency is preferable to the one introduced previously, because it will penalise an estimator if it has a large bias or a large variance or both. Notice that for an unbiased estimator the MSE and the variance are identical, so that the two measures of efficiency are identical if the estimators being compared are unbiased.

An important point to realise is that the quantities $\text{Bias}(\hat{\Theta})$, $\text{SE}(\hat{\Theta})$ and $\text{Eff}(\hat{\Theta}_1, \hat{\Theta}_2)$, can potentially depend on the value of the parameter θ. This means that the properties of an estimator may depend on the value of the parameter, and an estimator may have more desirable properties for some values of the parameter than for others.

Example 2.3 Returning to our prevalence example, recall that the mean of a $\text{Bin}(n, \theta)$ distribution is $n\theta$. Therefore the mean of our estimator $\hat{\Theta} = P$ is

$$\text{E}(\hat{\Theta}) = \frac{n\theta}{n} = \theta.$$

This means that our estimator in this example is an unbiased estimator of the unknown parameter. Since the variance of a $\text{Bin}(n, \theta)$ distribution is $n\theta(1 - \theta)$, the variance of our estimator is

$$\text{Var}(\hat{\Theta}) = \frac{n\theta(1 - \theta)}{n^2} = \frac{\theta(1 - \theta)}{n}.$$

Notice that this variance, and hence the standard error of our estimator, depends on the value of θ. This means that the estimator is more variable for some values of θ than for others. In fact, it can be shown that this estimator is most variable when $\theta = 0.5$, and least variable when θ is close to 0 or 1. Thus, its efficiency relative to some other possible estimator may also depend on the value of θ. In this example we will not compare our estimator with any other estimators in terms of efficiency, but this will be taken up in the extended example and the exercises later in the chapter. However, notice that

$$I(\theta)^{-1} = \text{E}\left[\frac{Y}{\theta^2} + \frac{n-Y}{(1-\theta)^2}\right]^{-1} = \frac{\theta(1-\theta)}{n} = \text{Var}(\hat{\Theta}),$$

meaning that our estimator in this example attains the minimum variance bound and is therefore the most efficient of all unbiased estimators. Notice also that as the sample size n becomes larger, the variance of our estimator becomes smaller, and will approach zero. This is an important property of an estimator and will now be discussed further.

2.6   Large sample properties

Much of statistical inference is based on large sample, or **asymptotic**, properties of estimation and testing procedures, which usually simplifies the study of such procedures. By large sample properties, we mean characteristics of the procedure that apply when the sample size tends to infinity. In practice of course we never have "infinite" sample size, but if the sample size is "large" then the asymptotic results will often provide an adequate approximation for our finite sample size. With this in mind we consider a number of large sample properties of estimators.

An essential property of a useful estimator is that as the sample size tends to infinity the estimate should be close to the true parameter value, eventually becoming identical to this value. This intuitive notion reflects an important statistical property of estimators that is referred to as consistency. An estimator $\hat{\Theta}$ is said to be a **consistent estimator** of a parameter θ if $\hat{\Theta}$ converges in probability to θ, written

$$\hat{\Theta} \xrightarrow{p} \theta \qquad \text{as } n \longrightarrow \infty.$$

Convergence in probability, which was introduced in Chapter 1, means that no matter how strictly we define "close", the probability of the estimator being close to the parameter value converges to 1 as the sample size tends to infinity. In other words, for any $\varepsilon > 0$ no matter how small,

$$\text{Pr}\left(|\hat{\Theta} - \theta| < \varepsilon\right) \longrightarrow 1 \qquad \text{as } n \longrightarrow \infty.$$

The above discussion provides a precise probabilistic definition of a consistent estimator. In practice, however, we often make use of more convenient conditions that are easier to verify and that guarantee the above definition of consistency is met. Consider the following two properties of an estimator $\hat{\Theta}$ as the sample size n becomes large:

$$\lim_{n\to\infty} \text{E}(\hat{\Theta}) = \theta \qquad \text{and} \qquad \lim_{n\to\infty} \text{Var}(\hat{\Theta}) = 0.$$

These two properties are highly desirable properties of estimators and help to reinforce what is meant by consistency. Firstly, observe that although these conditions do not require that an estimator be unbiased, they do require that in large samples it becomes unbiased, sometimes referred to as **asymptotically unbiased**. Secondly, observe that these conditions imply that in large samples the variability of the estimator diminishes until it eventually disappears. Thus, when taken together, these conditions would seem to say that the estimator will eventually coincide exactly with the true parameter value in large samples. In fact, it is a theorem of probability theory that if these two conditions hold then the above definition of consistency is met.

Consistency is important from the point of view of estimation of the unknown parameter, however, inferences about the parameter require the probability distribution of the estimator. While this distribution is usually quite complicated, often it is the case that in large samples the distribution of an estimator can be approximated by a normal distribution. This large sample normality greatly simplifies the process of making inferences about the parameter. For estimators that can be expressed as a mean, large sample normality follows from the Central Limit Theorem discussed in Chapter 1, which implies that the distribution of a mean is approximately normal in large samples. In fact, as we will discuss in Chapter 4, large sample normality applies much more broadly than this. In practice, a wide range of important estimators, many of which cannot be expressed as a mean, satisfy large sample normality.

Formally, large sample normality can be expressed using the probabilistic concepts of convergence in distribution and asymptotic normality. A consistent estimator $\hat{\Theta}$ of a parameter θ, is defined to have an **asymptotic normal distribution** if

$$\frac{\hat{\Theta} - \theta}{\sqrt{V(\theta)/n}} \xrightarrow{d} N(0,1) \qquad \text{as } n \to \infty$$

for some quantity $V(\theta)$. Convergence in distribution, specified by the notation $\xrightarrow{d}$, has a precise probabilistic meaning that we introduced in Chapter 1. In this case it means that the cumulative distribution function of the left-hand side converges to the cumulative distribution function of a standard normal random variable. For practical purposes, when a consistent estimator has an asymptotic normal distribution we can use this probabilistic interpretation to provide an approximate distribution in large samples, as we now describe.

In practice, asymptotic normality means that in large samples an estimator $\hat{\Theta}$ will have a distribution that is approximately normal with mean θ and variance $V(\theta)/n$, denoted

$$\hat{\Theta} \overset{d}{\approx} N\left(\theta, \frac{V(\theta)}{n}\right) \qquad \text{for large } n.$$

As long as we can identity the form of $V(\theta)$, large sample normality simplifies and unifies our approach to conducting inferences about the unknown parameter θ. In the next section we will describe how it can be used for the construction of confidence intervals, and in later chapters we will describe how it can be used for testing hypotheses about θ.

In Section 2.5 we discussed the minimum variance bound, which provides the smallest possible variance of an unbiased estimator. This result is also relevant for biased estimators in large samples, in that any estimator that is consistent and has an asymptotic variance that satisfies this lower bound has the smallest possible asymptotic variance. We refer to such estimators as **asymptotically efficient**. For consistent estimators, the quantity

$$\lim_{n\to\infty} \frac{I(\theta)^{-1}}{\text{Var}(\hat{\Theta})}$$

is referred to as the **asymptotic efficiency**. Clearly, an asymptotically efficient estimator has an asymptotic efficiency of 1, and is the best estimator in large samples.

As noted at the beginning of this chapter, for ease of presentation we have been assuming that we have just one parameter. In practice we may have more than one parameter, as exemplified in the extended example later in this chapter. When there is more than one parameter then analogous properties hold, however, the asymptotic variance becomes an asymptotic variance-covariance matrix, and the lower bound for the asymptotic variance involves taking a matrix inverse rather than a reciprocal. We will not discuss this further here, but will return to it in Chapter 4.

Example 2.4 In Example 2.3 we noted that the prevalence estimator $\hat{\Theta} = P$ is unbiased and has a variance that approaches zero as the sample size approaches infinity. Thus, $\hat{\Theta} = P$ is a consistent estimator of the population prevalence θ, and eventually coincides with the population prevalence as the sample size approaches infinity. We also saw in Example 2.3 that the prevalence estimator is an efficient estimator, in the sense that it attains the minimum variance bound. Clearly then, it will also be asymptotically efficient. Furthermore, as discussed in Chapter 1 and Example 2.3, the Central Limit Theorem implies that $\hat{\Theta}$ has an asymptotic normal distribution with $V(\theta) = \theta(1-\theta)$. That is, the distribution of $\hat{\Theta}$ can be approximated by a $N(\theta, \theta(1-\theta)/n)$ distribution when n is large.

2.7 Interval estimation

The observed value $\hat{\theta}$ of the estimator provides a single best value with which to estimate the unknown parameter θ, and is referred to as a **point estimate**. However, for more detailed inference about θ we require more than a single point estimate. We have already discussed the notion of estimator variability as a measure of the accuracy of an estimator. In this section we extend the use of estimator variability, as measured by the standard error, to provide us with an interval of parameter values that are in some sense "supported" by the sample. This allows us to conduct more detailed inference than a single point estimate would allow, and gives us information about the level of trust we should place in the point estimate.

From an intuitive point of view, an **interval estimate** is a range of parameter values within which we are "confident" that the true unknown value of θ lies. Another way of thinking about it is that the interval estimate includes all those parameter values that we would consider plausible, based on what we have observed in the sample.

The point estimate is in some sense the most plausible value, but the interval estimate contains a range of values that are also plausible.

This leads us to the concept of a **confidence interval**, which is the most common type of interval estimate. To define a confidence interval we first need to specify a **confidence level**, which expresses the extent of confidence that we wish to associate with our interval estimate. Often the confidence level is chosen to be 95%, but more generally we can specify the confidence level as $100(1-\alpha)\%$. Thus, different choices of α will produce different confidence levels, with $\alpha = 0.05$ corresponding to 95%.

Having specified the confidence level by choosing α, a $100(1-\alpha)\%$ confidence interval is then defined as any interval $[g(y), h(y)]$ where g and h are statistics that satisfy

$$\Pr[g(Y) \le \theta \le h(Y)] = 1 - \alpha.$$

Here the probability statement is made using the distribution of our sample Y.

We will return to the interpretation of a confidence interval in the next section, and discuss a common misinterpretation. However, before this we need to address the question of how to determine g and h, which are required to calculate the confidence interval. While there are a variety of ways to do this, it is most straightforward when our estimator is normally distributed, or is asymptotically normally distributed and the sample size is large. In this case,

$$\hat{\Theta} \overset{d}{\approx} N\left(\theta, \mathrm{SE}(\hat{\Theta})^2\right)$$

and the properties of the normal distribution lead to

$$\Pr\left[\hat{\Theta} - z_{1-\alpha/2} \times \mathrm{SE}(\hat{\Theta}) \le \theta \le \hat{\Theta} + z_{1-\alpha/2} \times \mathrm{SE}(\hat{\Theta})\right] = 1 - \alpha$$

where z_x is the x-percentile of the standard normal distribution. This would appear to provide us with a way of calculating a confidence interval, since the probability statement seems to be of the same form as that used above to define a confidence interval. However, in practice a complication arises from the fact that $\mathrm{SE}(\hat{\Theta})$ may depend on θ, whereas the quantities g and h are statistics that depend only on the sample. This can be overcome by defining an observed version of the standard error, called the estimated standard error $\mathrm{se}(\hat{\theta})$, which is the value of $\mathrm{SE}(\hat{\Theta})$ when it is evaluated at the sample estimate $\hat{\theta}$. Then estimating $\mathrm{SE}(\hat{\Theta})$ by $\mathrm{se}(\hat{\theta})$ in the above probability statement leads to

$$\Pr\left[\hat{\Theta} - z_{1-\alpha/2} \times \mathrm{se}(\hat{\theta}) \le \theta \le \hat{\Theta} + z_{1-\alpha/2} \times \mathrm{se}(\hat{\theta})\right] \approx 1 - \alpha$$

and an approximate $100(1-\alpha)\%$ confidence interval can be calculated as

$$\hat{\theta} \pm z_{1-\alpha/2} \times \mathrm{se}(\hat{\theta}).$$

The form of the above confidence interval shows the important role that the standard error plays in determining our range of plausible parameter values. In particular,

TABLE 2.1

95% confidence intervals for the population
prevalence (%)

p	$n = 100$	$n = 1000$	$n = 10000$
0.05	0.7 – 9.3	3.6 – 6.4	4.6 – 5.4
0.10	4.1 – 15.9	8.1 – 11.9	9.4 – 10.6
0.25	16.5 – 33.5	22.3 – 27.7	24.2 – 25.8
0.50	40.2 – 59.8	46.9 – 53.1	49.0 – 51.0

a smaller standard error will produce a narrower confidence interval, so more efficient estimators will tend to produce narrower confidence intervals. Furthermore, as
we shall see in the next example, because the standard error decreases as the sample
size increases, larger sample sizes also tend to produce narrower confidence intervals.

Example 2.5 From our discussion in Example 2.4, we know that the prevalence
estimator $\hat{\Theta} = P = Y/n$ has an asymptotic normal distribution with mean equal to
the population prevalence θ, and variance equal to $\theta(1 - \theta)/n$. We can therefore use
the normal distribution to calculate our confidence interval, assuming that we have
a "large" sample. However, as alluded to above, the standard error of our estimator,
$SE(\hat{\Theta}) = \sqrt{\theta(1 - \theta)/n}$, depends on the parameter we are trying to estimate and
therefore cannot be evaluated. We therefore need to approximate it by the estimated
standard error, $se(\hat{\theta}) = \sqrt{p(1 - p)/n}$, where $\hat{\theta} = p = y/n$ is our sample estimate.
Having done this we arrive at the 95% confidence interval

$$p \pm 1.96\sqrt{p(1 - p)/n}.$$

Thus, if our prevalence sample consists of $n = 1000$ individuals, of whom $y = 121$
have the disease, then $p = 0.121$ and a 95% confidence interval for the population
prevalence θ is the interval from 10.1% to 14.1%. Table 2.1 shows how our 95%
confidence interval would vary for different values of the sample prevalence and
different sample sizes. The first point to notice is that, for any given value of p, the
width of the confidence interval decreases as the sample size increases. This reflects
the fact that we have more confidence in the sample prevalence if it is obtained from
a larger sample. The second point to notice is that for any given sample size, the
confidence interval is narrower for values of p that are further away from 0.5. This
reflects the fact that the standard error depends on the prevalence, and is consistent
with our discussion in Example 2.3.

An important assumption of these confidence interval calculations is that the sample is large enough for the normal approximation to the binomial distribution to be
accurate. A common rule of thumb for defining "large" in the present context is
$n \geq 20/p$, which is satisfied by the calculations displayed in Table 2.1. If the normal
approximation is not accurate, then more complicated methods are needed based on
the exact binomial distribution. In Chapter 8 we will touch on these exact methods of

inference and return to this example to see how the approximate and exact methods compare.

2.8 Coverage probability

Although confidence intervals have a non-rigorous interpretation as a range of plausible parameter values, their formal definition is often more difficult to understand. Under the frequentist interpretation of probability, to correctly interpret a confidence interval one needs to imagine a hypothetical scenario in which we repeatedly take random samples from the population of interest. Each of these hypothetical repeated samples needs to be an identical replication of the random sampling process we used in our original observed sample. If we were to undertake this hypothetical sampling a large number of times, then our confidence interval definition implies that $100(1 - \alpha)\%$ of our samples will have confidence intervals that cover the true parameter value θ. That is, a confidence interval is a range of values that has been calculated in such a way that if the calculation is repeated on a large number of samples, the percentage of confidence intervals that cover the true parameter value will be equal to the desired confidence level.

The percentage of repeated samples that have confidence intervals covering the true parameter value is referred to as the **coverage probability**. For a valid confidence interval, the coverage probability should be equal to the desired confidence level. By choosing a high coverage probability, or equivalently a high confidence level, we then have a justification for using the confidence interval as an interval estimate. In particular, since we know the procedure will lead to an interval that covers the true parameter value in most samples (for example 95% of samples), we can therefore be confident that it includes the true parameter value when applied to our particular sample. In the next example we will illustrate the concept of a coverage probability, which underlies a rigorous understanding of a confidence interval.

Example 2.6 To illustrate the concept of a coverage probability, suppose that a prevalence sample of size $n = 1000$ is taken from a population with prevalence $\theta = 0.15$. The coverage probability describes how the confidence interval will behave in repeated sampling from this population. Figure 2.1 plots the 95% confidence intervals for 10 such repeated samples, each of size $n = 1000$. It is seen that for some samples the 95% confidence interval contains the population prevalence while for others it does not. In this case 8 out of 10 studies yielded a confidence interval that covers the true population prevalence of 15%. In the long run, if we repeated this sampling a very large number of times, 95% of samples would lead to a confidence interval that covers the population prevalence. In other words, the coverage probability is 0.95. As in Example 2.5, an important assumption here is that the normal approximation is accurate, which it is in this case. If it were not, then the actual coverage probability might not be 0.95. This would mean that the 95% confidence interval is not behaving the way it is supposed to behave and an exact method that does have a coverage probability of 0.95, such as that discussed in Chapter 8, should be used.

A common misinterpretation of a confidence interval is that it is an interval within which the population parameter value lies with probability $1 - \alpha$. Using our disease prevalence example in which we calculated a 95% confidence interval of 10.1% to 14.1%, this misinterpretation would involve claiming that "the probability that the population prevalence is between 10.1% and 14.1% is 0.95". From a frequentist perspective this is incorrect because the population prevalence is a fixed constant. Thus, either it is between 10.1% and 14.1% or it is not, and the probability that it lies in this interval is either 1 or 0 (we do not know which because the population prevalence is unknown). In general, probability statements about parameters are not meaningful within the frequentist paradigm. To correctly interpret a confidence interval we must think in terms of a coverage probability in repeated samples, as described above.

The fact that the precise interpretation of a confidence interval is often misunderstood, leads some statisticians to prefer an alternative approach to interval estimation which is based on Bayesian statistics. Under this approach, probability is interpreted as a degree of belief rather than a long-run frequency, and it is valid to make probability statements with respect to parameters. Thus, a statement such as "the probability that the population prevalence lies in the range 10.1% to 14.1% is 0.95" makes sense within the Bayesian paradigm, and reflects our degree of belief concerning the population prevalence. Most of this book is concerned with the more widely used frequentist approach, but we will provide a discussion of the Bayesian approach in Chapter 7.

2.9   Towards hypothesis testing

By providing a range of supported values for the parameter, a confidence interval also implicitly tells us which values are not supported by the sample – those values that are not in the confidence interval. This means that confidence intervals provide us with a way to make inferences about the parameter. For example, in Example 2.5, if we had started with an hypothesis that the population prevalence θ is no more than 5%, and we obtained a confidence interval ranging from 10.1% to 14.1%, we could reject that hypothesis because values of 5% or less are not supported by the data. One way of interpreting this is that the confidence interval contains all values θ_0 for which we would not be prepared to reject the hypothesis $\theta = \theta_0$. Conversely, all values θ_0 that are not contained in the confidence interval are values for which we would be prepared to reject the hypothesis $\theta = \theta_0$. This illustrates the intimate relationship between confidence intervals and hypothesis testing, and we will explore this further in subsequent chapters.

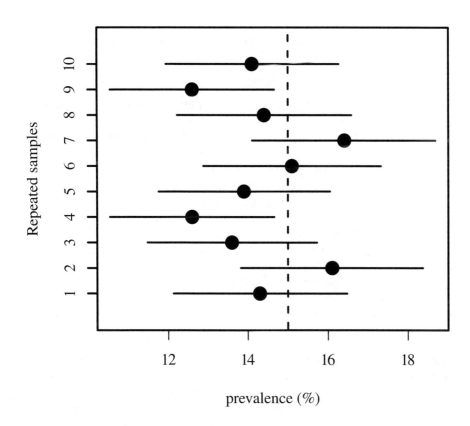

FIGURE 2.1
Sample prevalence and 95% confidence intervals for 10 samples of size 1000 from a
population with prevalence 15%

2.10 Extended example

The objective of this extended example is to review the estimation concepts introduced in this chapter. We will use the illustrative context of modelling a continuous
risk factor, cholesterol level, and compare different estimation approaches using concepts such as bias and efficiency. Most of what we discuss will be based on a parametric model that assumes cholesterol level has a normal distribution. However, we
will go on to highlight the importance of choosing an estimator that is appropriate
for the particular parametric model being used, by considering similar comparisons
under the assumption that the risk factor has a non-normal distribution.

2.10.1 Modelling cholesterol levels

There are many reasons why it might be of interest to model a risk factor, such as
cholesterol level, in a particular population. As an example, suppose that we are interested in designing a study that will compare two cholesterol-lowering treatments.
A typical design for such a study would involve screening potential participants and
enrolling those patients who have "high" cholesterol. If our study design involves enrolling 1000 participants with high cholesterol, then for resource planning we might
be interested in how many people we will need to screen to find 1000 people with
high cholesterol. This would require us to have information about the cholesterol
levels of people in the population that our screenees will be taken from, and in particular, the proportion of this population that has a cholesterol level in excess of the
cut-off that we define as "high". For concreteness, suppose that we are specifically
concerned with answering the following question: how many people would we need
to screen to obtain 1000 people with high cholesterol, if "high" is defined as a level
exceeding the following, when measured in millimoles per litre (mmol/L): (a) 5.5;
(b) 6.0; (c) 6.5; or (d) 7.0?

We will return to this question at the end of this section to provide answers.
Before we can do this, the first thing we need to do is develop a model for how
cholesterol level varies in the population from which we will screen our potential
participants. Figure 2.2 displays a sample of 100 cholesterol levels of people chosen
at random from the same population as those that will be screened for our future
cholesterol-lowering study. The first point to notice is that, at least visually, the normal distribution seems to be a reasonable model for the distribution of cholesterol
levels. There are more detailed ways of assessing whether a sample is approximately
normal, but for now suppose that we have decided to model the distribution of cholesterol levels using the normal distribution. We will return to the importance of this
decision later in the example.

Based on the normal distribution, we now have a parametric model that says the
cholesterol level X of a randomly chosen person has probability density function

$$f_X(x; \theta) = \frac{1}{\sqrt{2\pi\sigma^2}} \exp\left\{ -\frac{(x-\mu)^2}{2\sigma^2} \right\}$$

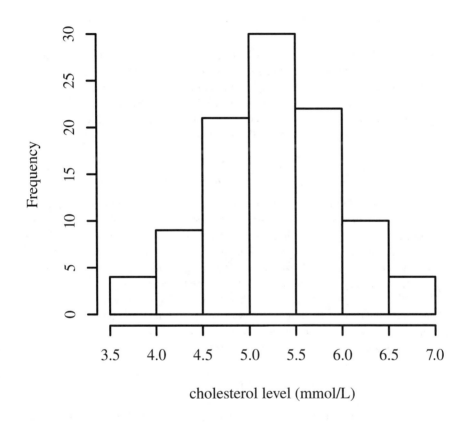

FIGURE 2.2
Histogram of the cholesterol levels for 100 individuals, showing an approximate normal distribution

where $\theta = (\mu, \sigma^2)$ is the (2-dimensional) parameter. Once we have estimated μ and σ^2 this distribution will be completely specified and we can answer our earlier question. We therefore need to decide how best to estimate μ and σ^2.

2.10.2   Estimating the parameters

Based on the normal model, our sample of $n = 100$ cholesterol levels $Y = (Y_1, \ldots, Y_n)$ has a joint probability density function

$$f_Y(y; \theta) = \prod_{i=1}^{n} f_i(y_i; \theta) = \left(\frac{1}{2\pi\sigma^2}\right)^{\frac{n}{2}} \exp\left\{-\sum_{i=1}^{n} \frac{(y_i - \mu)^2}{2\sigma^2}\right\}.$$

In subsequent chapters we will discuss how to use this joint distribution to motivate estimators of the unknown parameters. For now, we simply note that an obvious estimator of the population mean μ is the sample mean $\overline{Y}$. Based on the properties of expectations and variances, it is straightforward to show that $E(\overline{Y}) = \mu$ and $\text{Var}(\overline{Y}) = \sigma^2/n$. Furthermore, because sums of normal random variables are also normal, we know that the sampling distribution of this estimator is

$$\overline{Y} \overset{d}{=} N\left(\mu, \frac{\sigma^2}{n}\right).$$

The first point to note in relation to this sampling distribution is that, for estimating μ, the estimator has the property of being unbiased. The second point to note is that as n approaches infinity, the variance of the above normal distribution approaches 0. Thus, the estimator $\overline{Y}$ is a consistent estimator of μ, in that it will become closer and closer and eventually coincide with μ as n gets larger and larger. The next issue to address is whether an alternative to $\overline{Y}$ might be a better estimator.

We will consider one alternative estimator, the sample median M. Unlike for the sample mean, the exact sampling distribution of M is somewhat complicated. However, an important result from theoretical statistics tells us that the sample median has an approximate normal distribution for large n

$$M \overset{d}{\approx} N\left(\mu, \frac{\sigma^2 \pi}{2n}\right).$$

The first point to note from this result is that the asymptotic distribution of M has mean μ. That is, M is asymptotically unbiased. The second point to note is that, like for the sample mean, the variance of the sample median approaches 0 as the sample size gets larger. Thus, like the sample mean, the sample median is a consistent estimator of μ and will eventually coincide with μ as the sample size gets larger. Since both of our prospective estimators satisfy the minimal condition of consistency, the next step is to compare them based on their efficiency for estimating μ.

Although we have been focussing on estimating μ, recall that there are two parameters in the normal distribution. The obvious estimator of the variance σ^2 is the sample variance. We shall leave a study of this estimator to the exercises, where we will compare it with other possible estimators of σ^2.

2.10.3 Efficiency

Based on our definition of efficiency, and the variances of our estimators, the large sample efficiency of the sample median relative to the sample mean is

$$\text{Eff}(M, \overline{Y}) = \frac{\sigma^2/n}{\sigma^2 \pi/2n} = \frac{2}{\pi} = 0.64.$$

Thus, the sample median is only 64% as efficient as the sample mean for estimating μ in large samples, and this would lead us to prefer the sample mean over the sample median, at least in large samples when the normal distribution is an appropriate model. It is instructive to study this theoretical property empirically by considering how the two estimators behave in repeated samples of cholesterol levels.

Suppose we were able to undertake a large number of studies where for each study we sampled $n = 100$ people from the population and measured their cholesterol level. This would lead to a large number of estimates of μ based on the sample mean and the sample median. A comparison of the collection of estimates based on the sample mean, with the collection of estimates based on the sample median, allows us to investigate the relative efficiency of the two estimators empirically. Figure 2.3 shows the simulated results of such a repeated series of studies, in this case 1000 such studies. It has been assumed in these simulations that the population mean cholesterol level is 5.0 mmol/L and the population variance cholesterol level is 0.5 mmol/L. Figure 2.3 includes a histogram of the difference between the mean and the median in each study, as well as boxplots showing the range of the mean and median, respectively. In the latter case, the box in the middle of the plot provides the interquartile range and median of each set of estimates.

The first point to note from the histogram in Figure 2.3 is that the mean and the median have a difference that averages approximately zero over the 1000 studies. However, for individual studies the difference between the two estimates can range anywhere from approximately -0.2 to $+0.2$. Based on the boxplots, the distribution of both estimators looks fairly symmetric, which is consistent with our expectation that the estimators have approximate normal distributions. Importantly, the range over which the sample mean is spread is a little less than the range based on the sample median, indicating greater accuracy of the sample mean. Indeed, the variance of the 1000 estimates based on the sample mean is 0.0053 while the variance of the 1000 estimates based on the sample median is 0.0082. The ratio of these two variances, $0.0053/0.0082 = 0.65$, provides an empirical approximation to the theoretical efficiency that we derived above, and is quite close to the theoretical value 0.64.

Since our theoretical and simulation results indicate that the sample mean is a preferred estimator to the sample median in the present context, the natural question is whether there is another estimator that might be better than the sample mean. Based on the joint distribution of our sample Y, displayed above, it is possible to show that the variance of the sample mean is identical to the minimum variance bound discussed in Section 2.5. That is, the asymptotic efficiency of the sample mean is equal to 1, and no other consistent estimator can be more efficient than the sample mean in large samples, when the distribution of our cholesterol levels is normal. In

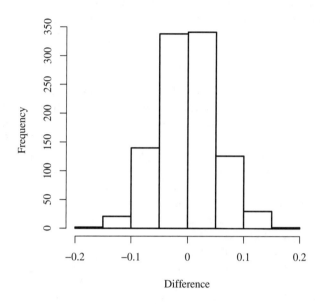

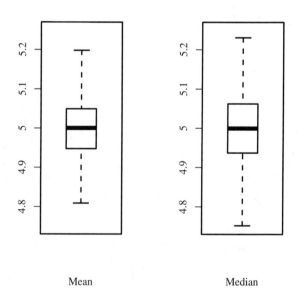

FIGURE 2.3
Histogram of the difference between the mean and the median in 1000 studies, and boxplots showing the range, interquartile range and median of the two sets of estimates

fact, it can be shown that the sample mean has a variance that is identical to the lower bound even in small samples, so there is no other unbiased estimator that has a variance smaller than the sample mean for small or large samples. These claims will be studied further in the exercises.

2.10.4 Standard errors and confidence intervals

The practical consequence of our choice of the sample mean over the sample median as our estimator of the population mean cholesterol level μ, is that our conclusion about this population parameter will be more precise. In particular, suppose we adopt as our estimate of the other parameter σ^2, the sample variance, $\hat{\sigma}^2 = s_{n-1}^2$. This is studied and justified in more detail in the exercises. Then our estimate of standard error when using the sample mean and sample median, respectively, will be

$$\mathrm{se}(\bar{y}) = \frac{s_{n-1}}{\sqrt{n}} \quad \text{and} \quad \mathrm{se}(m) = s_{n-1}\sqrt{\frac{\pi}{2n}}.$$

In the case of our sample of $n = 100$ cholesterol levels displayed in Figure 2.2, where $s_{n-1}^2 = 0.48$, this leads to standard errors of 0.069 and 0.087. Thus, given our observed estimates of $\bar{y} = 5.26$ and $m = 5.25$, the corresponding 95% confidence intervals for the population mean cholesterol level are

$$\bar{y} \pm 1.96 \frac{s_{n-1}}{\sqrt{n}} = (5.12, 5.40)$$

$$m \pm 1.96 s_{n-1}\sqrt{\frac{\pi}{2n}} = (5.08, 5.42).$$

Thus, while both methods lead to similar estimates in this sample, our confidence concerning the range of plausible values for the population mean, as reflected in the width of the confidence interval, is greater when using the sample mean.

Now that we have settled upon estimates of μ and σ^2, we are in a position to complete the task of estimating how many people we will need to screen to find 1000 people with high cholesterol. Based on the estimated distribution, $N(5.26, 0.48)$, the probability that a randomly chosen person will have high cholesterol, where high cholesterol is defined as a level in excess of c mmol/L, is given by

$$1 - \Phi\left(\frac{c - \hat{\mu}}{\hat{\sigma}}\right) = 1 - \Phi\left(\frac{c - 5.26}{0.69}\right).$$

Thus, dividing 1000 by the above estimate for any assumed value of c, yields the average number of people that will need to be screened and allows us to answer the question we posed at the beginning of this example, as summarised in Table 2.2. It can be seen that, while lower values of the cut-off for high cholesterol are likely to lead to a feasible number of screenings, choosing higher values to define high cholesterol would require extremely large numbers of patients to be screened and may well be infeasible. Such information would be important to take into account in designing the study that we described earlier.

TABLE 2.2
Screenings to identify 1000 people with high
cholesterol (mmol/L)

Cut-point	5.5	6.0	6.5	7.0
Screenings	2,748	7,055	27,656	171,268

2.10.5   Departures from normality

In this example we used a histogram of our sample to motivate a model based on the normal distribution. It is important to remember that our assessment of different estimators relates to this particular model and may not hold for data that follow other models. In particular, if the data come from a non-normal distribution, it is possible that the sample median may perform as well or better than the sample mean. To see an example of this consider a repeat of the simulation study in Figure 2.3, with the exception that the cholesterol levels will be sampled from a non-normal distribution. The non-normal distribution we shall use is one that models "outliers" in the data. That is, we will assume that cholesterol levels in the population have the same normal distribution as was assumed for Figure 2.3, however, for $k\%$ of individuals the cholesterol level is recorded incorrectly as an arbitrary value distributed randomly between zero and 10 mmol/L (i.e. according to a uniform distribution). Since the sample median is less sensitive to extreme values than the sample mean, it is plausible that it may have better properties for such data. This is borne out in Table 2.3, which shows the effect of such "contamination" of the normal distribution on the relative efficiency of the two estimators, for increasing values of k. Here, the efficiency is the ratio of the variances of the sample mean to the sample median in a series of 1000 repeated studies of sample size 100.

The above example demonstrates that, while being superior when the cholesterol levels are normally distributed, the sample mean becomes inferior to the sample median when observations arise that are extreme relative to the normal distribution. It highlights the importance of identifying an appropriate model for the data, prior to determining appropriate estimators of the unknown population parameters, and demonstrates that an estimator that is optimal for one model may not retain its optimality if the assumed model is not satisfied. In this book we will often focus on the performance of estimation and inference methods assuming that an appropriate model has been identified. However, it should be remembered that identifying the right model in the first place is not always easy and is a key aspect of applied biostatistics.

TABLE 2.3

Simulated efficiency of the median relative to
the mean with contamination

Contamination	0%	1%	5%	10%
Efficiency		0.65	0.73	1.04	1.37

Exercises

1. In the extended example we focused on estimation of μ, the population mean cholesterol level. Now consider estimation of σ^2, the variance of cholesterol levels in the population. The following are two possible estimators of σ^2, which are alternative versions of the sample variance, and differ only by whether we divide by $n-1$ or n:

$$S_{n-1}^2 = \frac{1}{n-1} \sum_{i=1}^{n} (Y_i - \overline{Y})^2 = \frac{1}{n-1} \sum_{i=1}^{n} Y_i^2 - \frac{n}{n-1} \overline{Y}^2$$

and

$$S_n^2 = \frac{1}{n} \sum_{i=1}^{n} (Y_i - \overline{Y})^2 = \frac{1}{n} \sum_{i=1}^{n} Y_i^2 - \overline{Y}^2.$$

(a) Show that S_n^2 is a biased estimator of σ^2.

(b) Show that S_{n-1}^2 is an unbiased estimator of σ^2.

(c) Is S_n^2 asymptotically unbiased?

2. Consider another estimator of σ^2, based on the interquartile range of the sample. Let $Y_{(i)}$ be the ith smallest observation in the sample, or the ith "order statistic". Then the following is an alternative estimator of σ^2,

$$R^2 = \frac{1}{1.349^2} (Y_{(0.75n)} - Y_{(0.25n)})^2.$$

Note that if $0.25n$ or $0.75n$ are not integers then we use the largest integers not exceeding these numbers.

(a) What would be the advantage of using R^2 in preference to S_{n-1}^2?

(b) What would be a potential disadvantage of using R^2?

(c) If Y_i is normally distributed then $E(Y_{(pn)}) \to \mu + \sigma \Phi^{-1}(p)$ as $n \to \infty$, where $0 < p < 1$. In other words the expected value of the sample percentiles converge to the population percentiles. Use this fact to show that R is an asymptotically unbiased estimator of σ.

3. For this exercise you will need to use the simulation function `cnorm.sim` described in Appendix 2. Carry out a simulation of 1000 studies each involving observation of the cholesterol level of n individuals, for $n = 20, 50, 100$ and 1000 (so 4000 studies will need to be simulated overall). Assume that the cholesterol level in the population is normally distributed with mean 5.0 mmol/L and variance 0.5 mmol/L.

   (a) Calculate the mean and variance of the sampling distribution of the estimators R^2 and S^2_{n-1}, for each value of n.

   (b) Calculate the efficiency of R^2 relative to S^2_{n-1}, for each value of n.

   (c) Do R^2 and S^2_{n-1} appear to be consistent estimators of σ^2? Give reasons.

   (d) Which estimator would you prefer and why?

4. For this exercise you will need to do similar simulations as in Exercise 3, but with the addition of some non-normal observations to the samples, as we discussed in the extended example. For this exercise use a sample size of $n = 100$ for all questions.

   (a) Using the function `cnorm.sim`, carry out simulations identical to those in Exercise 3, for $n = 100$, with the exception that for $k\%$ of the sample the observation will be recorded incorrectly (for example due to laboratory errors) and will be uniformly distributed between 0 and 10. Use $k = 0\%, 1\%$ and 5%. Based on your simulations, calculate the mean, variance and bias of the two estimators for each value of k.

   (b) Using the results from part (a), calculate the efficiency of the two estimators for each value of k using (i) the variances and (ii) the mean squared errors. Which measure of efficiency do you think is more appropriate?

   (c) Draw conclusions about the relative merits of the two estimators assuming that cholesterol levels in the population are normally distributed when (i) measurements are always recorded correctly, and (ii) a small percentage of measurements is recorded incorrectly (potentially producing small or large outliers).

5. Suppose that cholesterol levels have a normal distribution and that the population variance is known to be $\sigma^2 = 1$.

   (a) Using the material in Sections 2.5 and 2.6, justify the claim made in Section 2.10.3 that the sample mean has the smallest possible asymptotic variance of any consistent estimator.

   (b) Is the sample mean the best possible unbiased estimator in small samples?

6. In a study of a new blood pressure lowering drug it was found that the mean reduction in systolic blood pressure was $\bar{y}$ with a standard deviation of s_{n-1}, each measured in millimetres of mercury (mmHg). Assume a parametric model for

this sample in which the reduction in systolic blood pressure for each patient has a normal distribution, $N(\mu, \sigma^2)$. Consider the following two 95% confidence intervals for the population mean reduction in systolic blood pressure on the drug

$$\bar{y} \pm z_{0.975} \frac{s_{n-1}}{\sqrt{n}} \quad \text{and} \quad \bar{y} \pm t_{n-1,0.975} \frac{s_{n-1}}{\sqrt{n}}$$

Here, n is the sample size and the percentiles of the normal and t_{n-1} distributions are given by the following table:

	$n = 10$	$n = 20$	$n = 40$	$n = 80$	$n = 160$
$z_{0.975}$	1.96	1.96	1.96	1.96	1.96
$t_{n-1,0.975}$	2.26	2.09	2.02	1.99	1.97

For this exercise you will need to use the simulation function cnorm.sim described in Appendix 2.

(a) Which of the two confidence intervals will have the largest coverage probability (give reasons without any calculations)?

(b) Suppose that the population mean reduction in systolic blood pressure is 10 mmHg and that the population standard deviation of the reduction in systolic blood pressure is 12 mmHg. Based on these assumptions about the population, for each of the sample sizes in the table use the function cnorm.sim to carry out a simulation of 1000 studies to obtain 1000 simulated sample means and sample variances. Use these simulated sample means and sample variances to calculate the two confidence intervals for each study. Hence estimate the coverage probability of each of the confidence intervals. An example of the R commands needed to do these calculations is given in Appendix 2.

(c) Based on your results in part (b), summarise under what circumstances the confidence intervals differ in their coverage probabilities, and which confidence interval you would prefer.

(d) Suppose that in a particular study with a sample size of 20 patients treated with the drug, we observed a sample mean reduction in systolic blood pressure of 6.1 mmHg and a sample standard deviation reduction of 13.1 mmHg. Does this sample provide evidence that the drug reduces blood pressure on average (give reasons)?

(e) The estimate $\bar{y}$ is the observed value of the estimator $\bar{Y}$. What is the expectation and variance of this estimator? Hence justify that the sample mean is an unbiased and consistent estimator of the population mean.

7. Suppose that two independent random samples of size n_1 and n_2 observations are selected from normal populations. Let $X_1, \ldots, X_{n_1}$ and $Y_1, \ldots, Y_{n_2}$ be the two random samples and suppose that $X_i \overset{d}{=} N(\mu_1, \sigma^2)$ and $Y_i \overset{d}{=} N(\mu_2, \sigma^2)$. Let S_X^2 and

S_Y^2 be the sample variances from the two samples, respectively, using the $n-1$ version of the sample variance defined in Exercise 1. Consider the following two possible estimators of the common variance σ^2

$$S_1^2 = \frac{(n_1-1)S_X^2 + (n_2-1)S_Y^2}{n_1+n_2-2} \quad \text{and} \quad S_2^2 = \frac{(S_X^2+S_Y^2)}{2}.$$

(a) Show that both estimators are unbiased estimators of σ^2.

(b) Using the relationship between the $\chi^2(1)$ and standard normal distributions, and properties of the $\chi^2(v)$ distribution, find $\text{Var}(S_1^2)$ and $\text{Var}(S_2^2)$.

(c) Derive the efficiency of the estimator S_2^2 relative to the S_1^2. When is the relative efficiency equal to 1?

(d) Show that both estimators are consistent estimators of σ^2.

(e) Which estimator would you prefer?

8. Review the discussion of disease incidence estimation in the exercises from Chapter 1. Recall the following notation: the sample cohort consists of n individuals of whom X experienced disease onset during the follow-up period; the average follow-up is $A = F/n$ years where F is the total person-years of follow-up; λ is the population incidence rate, that is, the rate of occurrence of new cases of the disease. The estimator of the incidence rate is $\hat{\Lambda} = X/F$ (we called this R in Chapter 1).

(a) Assuming that X has a Poisson distribution, show that $\hat{\Lambda}$ is an unbiased and consistent estimator of λ.

(b) Show that $\hat{\Lambda}$ attains the minimum variance bound for unbiased estimators of λ.

(c) Using the approximate normal distribution for $\hat{\Lambda}$, write down $\text{SE}(\hat{\Lambda})$ and its estimate $\text{se}(\hat{\lambda})$.

(d) Suppose we observed 350 individuals for an average of 5 years, and in that time 31 individuals developed the disease of interest. Provide an estimate and a 95% confidence interval for λ. As the rate is small, express your answer per 1000 years of follow-up.

(e) Is it plausible that the incidence rate is no greater than 15 events per 1000 years of follow-up?

9. In this exercise we consider an alternative confidence interval for the incidence rate λ from Exercise 8. Firstly, consider a Poisson random variable Y with mean θ. Then for large n, it can be shown that $\sqrt{Y}$ has an approximate $N(\sqrt{\theta}, 0.25)$ distribution.

(a) Use this result to write down an approximate 95% confidence interval for $\sqrt{\lambda}$, and hence an approximate 95% confidence interval for λ.

(b) Calculate this confidence interval for the sample described in Exercise 8(d) and compare your results.

10. Suppose the population we are studying has a population incidence rate of 15 events per 1000 years of follow-up, and our study design is such that we follow 350 individuals for an average of 5 years. Suppose that we repeated such a study 10 times on the same population. Using the function `inc.sim` described in Appendix 2, simulate the results of these 10 studies, and for each study calculate the sample incidence rate and both 95% confidence intervals described above.

   (a) What proportion of the confidence intervals include the population incidence rate?

   (b) Repeat part (a) using 1000 simulations and hence calculate and compare the coverage probabilities of the two confidence intervals.

   (c) Repeat part (b) supposing that we only followed 150 individuals for an average of 5 years.

3

Likelihood

In Chapter 2 we discussed parametric statistical models, and considered desirable properties of estimators of the unknown parameter. While we considered a number of criteria by which a given estimator can be judged, and discussed some particular estimators appropriate for specific models, we did not discuss approaches to identifying estimators in the first place. In this chapter we introduce the concept of likelihood, which is the basis of the most important general approach to parameter estimation. Our primary objective in this chapter is to present likelihood as a tool for identifying the level of support that the observed data provide for particular values of the unknown parameter. This will include a discussion of the likelihood function, together with the idea of data reduction and the concept of sufficiency. After a discussion of various extensions to multiple parameter contexts, the concepts will be illustrated using an extended example on disease incidence rates. The likelihood function as a tool for deriving estimation procedures will then be taken up in Chapter 4.

3.1 Statistical likelihood

In a parametric statistical model, likelihood may be thought of as the extent to which our sample provides support for particular values of the parameter. The notion of likelihood applies to values of the parameter, given a specific value for our sample. Thus, we may speak of the likelihood associated with a parameter value $\theta = \theta_0$, given an observed sample value $Y = y$. If the observed data provide more support for one value of the parameter than for another value, then the likelihood is higher for the former parameter value.

The way in which likelihood is defined is easiest to think about in the context of a discrete variable that is modelled by means of a discrete probability function. In this case the likelihood associated with the parameter value θ_0 is the probability that our sample Y would take the observed value y, assuming the true value of the parameter is θ_0. Thus, given our particular observed sample value y, the **likelihood** associated with the parameter value θ_0 is

$$L(\theta_0; y) = \Pr(Y = y \mid \theta = \theta_0) = f_Y(y; \theta_0).$$

The notation $\Pr(Y = y \mid \theta = \theta_0)$ means the probability of the event $Y = y$, under the assumption that $\theta = \theta_0$. Although this probability statement uses the same notation as a conditional probability, strictly speaking it is not a conditional probability because θ is a parameter not a random variable. Nonetheless, this type of notation is common in this context, and it is important to understand that it is a probability under an assumption about θ, rather than a true conditional probability.

Using the definition of likelihood, it can be seen that if a particular parameter value makes it relatively unlikely that we would have observed the sample that we did in fact observe, then the likelihood for that parameter value will be low relative to other parameter values. Parameter values that make the observed sample relatively likely, that is parameter values with high likelihood, are the values that we will consider to be supported by the data.

The likelihood associated with a particular parameter value is relevant for the particular sample that we have observed. If another sample had been observed, or if another study is carried out that yields a different sample, then the likelihood associated with that parameter value would be different. Likelihood is therefore a measure of support for parameter values given that we already have a sample. However, in order to understand likelihood, we need to imagine the circumstances prior to us taking this sample. We need to imagine what the probability was, prior to the study starting, of us ending up with the sample that we did in fact end up with. This probability corresponds to the likelihood and parameter values with high likelihood are those that make this probability high, based on the assumed parametric model.

While likelihood is easiest to conceptualise in the context of discrete variables where it corresponds to a probability, the same principle applies for continuous variables. In this case the likelihood is defined analogously to the discrete case described above,

$$L(\theta_0; y) = f_Y(y; \theta_0)$$

with the exception that f_Y now stands for the probability density function rather than the probability function. Thus, the likelihood corresponds to the probability density (rather than the probability) associated with the observed sample. Apart from the distinction between the probability density function and the probability function, calculations of the likelihood for specific parameter values are carried out in the same way for discrete and continuous models. Likelihood calculations for a discrete model are illustrated in the following example.

Example 3.1 As in previous chapters, the binomial distribution provides a convenient context in which to illustrate basic concepts in statistical inference, and we shall therefore return to the setting of a binomial prevalence study as an initial illustration of the concept of likelihood. Consider the disease prevalence study discussed in previous chapters, in which a sample of 1000 individuals are observed and it is found that 121 individuals have evidence of prior disease onset. We have already discussed the use of the sample prevalence $\hat{\theta} = 121/1000 = 12.1\%$ as an estimate of the population prevalence θ. It is instructive to consider what the likelihood associated with this value of the parameter would be, and to compare it with the likelihood for other values of the parameter. According to our definition of likelihood above, given the observation $y = 121$, the likelihood corresponding to a prevalence of 12.1% is

$$\begin{aligned} \Pr(Y = 121 \mid \theta = 0.121) &= f_Y(121; 0.121) \\ &= \frac{1000!}{879!121!} 0.121^{121} 0.879^{1000-121} = 0.0387 \end{aligned}$$

using the fact that Y has a $\mathrm{Bin}(1000, \theta)$ distribution. This value represents the probability, prior to the study starting, that we would observe the sample that we did end up observing, assuming the true value of the population prevalence is 12.1%. This may seem like a small value, but this is because there are so many (1001) possible outcomes that could have arisen. In fact, the absolute magnitude of the likelihood is largely irrelevant, and what we are most interested in is the relative magnitude of the likelihood for one parameter value compared to the likelihood for another parameter value. This allows us to identify the parameter values that have greatest support. Consider another possible value for the parameter, say 15.0%. To what extent is a population prevalence of 12.1% more supported by the data than a population prevalence of 15.0%? Using the same computational approach, the likelihood associated with the parameter value 15.0% is

$$\begin{aligned} \Pr(Y = 121 \mid \theta = 0.150) &= f_Y(121; 0.150) \\ &= \frac{1000!}{879!121!} 0.150^{121} 0.850^{1000-121} = 0.0012. \end{aligned}$$

This is less than the likelihood corresponding to a value of 12.1%, and so the parameter value 15.0% is less supported by the data. The relative magnitude of the two likelihoods may be quantified using their ratio, which in this case is

$$\frac{f_Y(121; 0.121)}{f_Y(121; 0.150)} = 32.88$$

which differs slightly from $0.0387/0.0012$ due to rounding. Roughly speaking, this calculation indicates that the level of support provided by the data for the value 12.1% is about 33 times greater than the level of support for the value 15.0%. Notice that if we are only concerned with the relative magnitude of the likelihood for different parameter values, then the factor $\frac{1000!}{879!121!}$ is irrelevant for our comparison, because it is common to both values and cancels out when we calculate the ratio. In general, as discussed further below, we can drop from the likelihood any common factor that does not depend on the parameter. Thus, in the present setting, the two likelihoods would be $0.121^{121} 0.879^{879}$ and $0.150^{121} 0.850^{879}$, respectively, and the relative magnitude would of course be unchanged at 32.88.

3.2 Likelihood function

Our discussion in the previous section focused on the comparison of the likelihood associated with two different parameter values. By considering the entire range of possible values of the likelihood, across all possible values of the parameter, the likelihood becomes a function of the parameter value. This function is referred to as the **likelihood function**, and is written as $L(\theta)$, or $L(\theta;y)$ if one wishes to emphasise that the function depends on the observed sample y. It is important to distinguish the roles of θ and y in the likelihood function, and to contrast this with their roles in the probability (density) function of the sample. The distinction between the likelihood function of the parameter and the probability (density) function of the sample is the perspective that one takes with regard to which quantity, θ or y, is the x-variable in the function. The likelihood function is a function of the parameter θ, that is θ is the x-variable, but it depends on the observed sample value y. Thus, for a particular value of the sample we would have a corresponding likelihood function of θ, while for another value of the sample we would have a different likelihood function of θ. On the other hand, the probability (density) function is a function of y, and depends on the parameter θ. Thus, for a particular value of the parameter we would have a corresponding probability (density) function of the sample y, while for another value of the parameter we would have a different probability (density) function of y.

Example 3.2 For the disease prevalence context discussed in Example 3.1, the likelihood function of the parameter and the probability function of the sample are written as

$$L(\theta;y) = f_Y(y;\theta) = \frac{1000!}{(1000-y)!y!}\theta^y(1-\theta)^{1000-y}$$

for $0 \le \theta \le 1$ and $y = 0, 1, \ldots, 1000$. To emphasise the distinction between the likelihood function of the parameter, and the probability function of the sample, we will first consider the above expression as a function of θ, and then consider it as function of y. Consider two different studies in which $y = 121$ and $y = 509$ diseased individuals were observed, respectively. Substituting these two values of y into the above expression leads to two different likelihood functions of θ corresponding to those samples. Figure 3.1 compares these two likelihood functions. Now consider two different assumptions about the population prevalence, namely $\theta = 12.1\%$ and $\theta = 50.9\%$, respectively. Substituting these two values of θ into the above expression leads to two different probability functions of y corresponding to those parameter values. Figure 3.1 compares these two probability functions, where values of y for which the probability function is zero have been omitted from the graph. A comparison of the top two graphs with the bottom two graphs makes the distinction between the likelihood function and the probability function apparent, the former being a function of θ (dependent on y) and the latter being a function of y (dependent on θ). Indeed in this case, the likelihood function is a continuous function, whereas the probability function is a discrete function. As an additional point, notice from the two likelihood functions that the observed sample y has a substantial effect on the resulting likelihood function. Importantly, it can be seen in both cases that the parameter value that is most supported by the data, or in other words the population prevalence value with the greatest likelihood, corresponds to the observed sample prevalence. In fact, this is a general result, and provides a theoretical basis for using the sample prevalence to estimate the population prevalence, as will be discussed further in Chapter 4.

As alluded to in Example 3.1, we are only interested in the relative magnitude of the likelihood for one parameter value compared to other parameter values. The absolute value of the likelihood for any particular parameter value has little meaning on its own. The relative magnitude of the likelihood corresponding to two different parameter values is measured using their ratio, referred to as a **likelihood ratio**. For this reason, the likelihood function only needs to be defined up to a proportionality factor that does not depend on the parameter θ. What we mean by this is that any function of θ that can be expressed as $f_Y(y;\theta)$ multiplied by a term that does not depend on θ can be used as the likelihood function. Thus, the likelihood function is defined as any function of θ that can be expressed as

$$L(\theta) = L(\theta;y) = c(y)f_Y(y;\theta).$$

This sometimes simplifies our study of the likelihood function as it means that superfluous terms can be dropped. It is the reason why, in Example 3.1, we were able to drop the multiplicative factor that does not depend on θ, and retain the identical conclusion with regard to the relative support that the data provide for the two parameter values under consideration.

3.3 Log-likelihood function

Since the likelihood function is always non-negative, it is possible to take its logarithm, $\ell(\theta) = \log L(\theta)$, which is referred to as the **log-likelihood function**. The log function is an increasing function so if one parameter value has a larger likelihood than another parameter value, it will always have a larger log-likelihood as well. This means that in terms of deciding whether one parameter value is more supported by the data than another parameter value, it does not matter whether we use the likelihoods associated with those parameter values, or the log-likelihoods. As discussed below, this property means that, when taken together with other desirable properties of the log-likelihood function, it is usual to use the log-likelihood rather than the likelihood. In all cases when we refer to the log we shall mean the natural logarithm (base e).

Recall that in the common situation that our sample corresponds to n independent observations $y = (y_1, \ldots, y_n)$, the joint probability (density) function is the product of the individual probability (density) functions, $f_i(y_i;\theta)$, associated with the individual observations. The likelihood function is therefore often a product of the form

$$L(\theta) = \prod_{i=1}^{n} f_i(y_i;\theta).$$

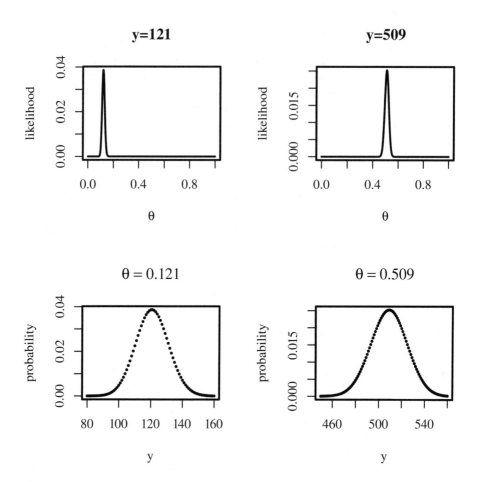

FIGURE 3.1
Likelihood functions and probability functions corresponding to various values of
the observed sample (y) and the population prevalence (θ)

Since the log of a product is the sum of the logs, this means that the log-likelihood is often a summation of the form

$$\ell(\theta) = \sum_{i=1}^{n} \log f_i(y_i; \theta)$$

which is often easier to study theoretically than the likelihood. For example, in Chapter 4 we will discuss methods for finding the most supported parameter estimate, which is often far more convenient using the summation form of the log-likelihood rather than the product form of the likelihood. Furthermore, the probabilistic properties of likelihoods and their ratios, which will be discussed later in this book, are easier to describe and are often more informative when expressed on the log scale. In view of this convenience, and because comparisons of the levels of support for different parameter values are not altered by whether we use the likelihood function or the log-likelihood function, it is more common to derive estimation and inference procedures using the log-likelihood function.

In the previous section we discussed the fact that multiplicative factors that do not depend on the parameter can be dropped from the likelihood function if we are using ratios of likelihoods to compare the relative levels of support for different parameter values. When using the log-likelihood function, rather than the likelihood function, we measure the relative levels of support for different parameter values using the difference of the log-likelihoods, rather than the ratio. This will be discussed in some detail when we come to discuss the use of log-likelihoods for hypothesis testing in Chapter 6. If we are concerned only with differences between log-likelihoods then we can drop additive terms that do not depend on θ since these terms will cancel out when we take differences. Thus, the log-likelihood function can be defined as any function of θ that can be expressed as

$$\ell(\theta) = \log L(\theta) = c(y) + \log f_Y(y; \theta).$$

Example 3.3 Returning to Example 3.2, the log-likelihood function is

$$\ell(\theta) = \log\left(\frac{1000!}{(1000-y)!y!}\right) + y\log(\theta) + (1000-y)\log(1-\theta)$$

where $0 \leq \theta \leq 1$ and $\log(0)$ is interpreted as $-\infty$. This leads to log-likelihood functions plotted in Figure 3.2, for the two samples discussed in Example 3.2. As expected, parameter values with high likelihood in Figure 3.1 also have high log-likelihood in Figure 3.2, and in particular, the observed sample prevalence provides the parameter value with the highest log-likelihood. Of course, the term "high" is meant relative to other parameter values, as the absolute value of the log-likelihood is not meaningful. According to our earlier discussion, there is no need to retain additive terms in the log-likelihood that do not depend on the parameter. Thus, it would be easier, and statistically equivalent, to use the following log-likelihood function,

$$\ell(\theta) = y\log(\theta) + (1000-y)\log(1-\theta)$$

which corresponds with the simpler likelihood function

$$L(\theta) = \theta^y (1-\theta)^{1000-y}.$$

In Example 3.2, we noted that the different sample values for y lead to substantially different likelihood functions. The same is of course true for log-likelihood functions, and notice in particular that the log-likelihood function corresponding to $y = 509$ is flatter, or less pointy, than the log-likelihood function for $y = 121$. This means that there is a wider range of parameter values with a log-likelihood value that is close to the value achieved by the most supported value, the sample prevalence. In other words, there is a wider range of parameter values that is supported by the data, which suggests that our confidence interval for the population prevalence should be wider when $y = 509$ than when $y = 121$. In Chapter 4 we will discuss further the fact that the curvature of the log-likelihood function, or in other words how flat it is, allows us to assess how uncertain our estimate is and determines the width of our confidence interval.

3.4   Sufficient statistics and data reduction

A statistical model involves postulating a probability distribution for our sample, which depends on a parameter that represents an important unknown characteristic in the population of interest. It is because the distribution of our sample depends on the parameter that we are able to use the sample to obtain information about the parameter. A sample cannot be used to obtain information about a characteristic of the population if the distribution of the sample does not depend on that characteristic. We will now take this idea one step further, and discuss how to identify aspects of the sample that contain all of the available information about the parameter.

In Chapter 2 we introduced the term statistic to represent any quantity that can be calculated from the sample, that is, any function of the sample that does not depend on θ. We used the notation $T = T(Y)$ for a statistic, with observed value $t = T(y)$, an example of which is the sum $\sum y_i$ of all the individual observations $y = (y_1, \ldots, y_n)$. The question of interest in this section is: when can we reduce our observed sample down to an observed statistic $T(y)$ and still retain all the information that the sample has to offer about the parameter θ? To answer this, consider a discrete model and consider the probability function of our sample, given that we know the observed value of the statistic, $T = t$. For example, the probability function of the sample given that we know the sum of all the observations in the sample. We call this a **conditional distribution**, and it is defined in terms of the conditional probability

$$f_{Y|T}(y \mid t) = \Pr(Y = y \mid T = t).$$

Then, the answer to our question is: when the above conditional distribution does not depend on θ. When the conditional distribution of the sample, given the value

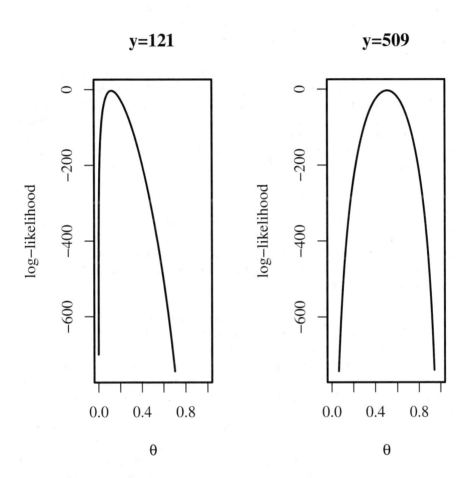

FIGURE 3.2
Log-likelihood functions for the population prevalence (θ) for two values of the observed sample (y)

of the statistic, does not depend on our parameter then the sample has no more information to offer us about the parameter over and above the information provided by the statistic. In this case the statistic is "sufficient" for conveying all the available information about the parameter, and is referred to as a **sufficient statistic**. Thus, for example, if the sum of the observations is a sufficient statistic then we do not need to know all of the individual observations in the sample, since we can extract all of the available information using only their sum. Although we limited our attention to discrete models above, a similar rationale applies to the conditional density function from a continuous model.

It turns out that there is a simple way to check whether a particular statistic is a sufficient statistic, and this method can be used for both continuous and discrete models. Suppose that the likelihood function for the full sample y is $L(\theta;y)$. If this likelihood function can be rearranged algebraically so that it can be written as the product of two terms, one term that depends only on y and not θ, and another term that depends on θ and some statistic $T(y)$, then this statistic is a sufficient statistic. That is, $T(y)$ is a sufficient statistic whenever the likelihood function can written as

$$L(\theta;y) = c(y)L^*(\theta;T(y))$$

for some functions c and L^*. If it is not possible to write the likelihood function in this way then the statistic $T(y)$ is not a sufficient statistic. This criterion is called the **factorisation criterion** for a sufficient statistic. It mirrors our previous discussion concerning dropping terms that do not depend on θ from the likelihood function. In the above expression, according to our earlier discussion, we are able to drop the term $c(y)$ and use $L^*(\theta;T(y))$ as our likelihood function. Thus, for statistical inference based on the likelihood function, we do not lose any information if we only know the value of $T(y)$ rather than the entire sample. In other words, the value of the sufficient statistic contains all the information available in the sample about the parameter.

Of course, an implicit assumption in the above discussion is that it is appropriate to base our inferences on the likelihood function. More specifically, we are effectively assuming that the likelihood function contains all the information in the sample concerning the parameter, otherwise it would not be appropriate to reduce the sample down to a sufficient statistic. This is an important assumption which is referred to as the **likelihood principle**. It is related to another implicit assumption that we have made in this chapter, which is that likelihood is the appropriate measure of the support that the sample has for a particular parameter value. More specifically, we have effectively been assuming that the likelihood ratio associated with two parameter values is all that is needed to determine which of the two parameter values is more supported by the sample. This assumption is called the **law of likelihood**. The appropriateness of these basic tenets of likelihood-based inference has generated much discussion and even controversy over the years. Such foundational issues will not occupy us further here, but texts on the foundations of statistics often take up these issues in great detail, see for example the books by Edwards (1992) and Royall (1997) as well as others referred to in Appendix 3. Our focus here, however, will be on less philosophical matters, beginning with an example of how to apply the factorisation criterion in practice.

Example 3.4 Consider the study discussed in the extended example of Section 2.10, which involved estimating the distribution of cholesterol levels in a particular population, using a parametric model based on the normal distribution. Suppose that we know that the variance of cholesterol levels in the population is 1.0. This is of course an unrealistic assumption in practice, but we will use it initially and then consider the more realistic situation of an unknown population variance in Example 3.5. Based on the probability density function that we wrote down in Section 2.10, with $\sigma^2 = 1.0$, the likelihood function corresponding to our sample of cholesterol levels $y = (y_1, \ldots, y_n)$ is as follows, where $T(y) = \sum_{i=1}^{n} y_i$

$$
\begin{aligned}
L(\mu) &= \left(\frac{1}{2\pi}\right)^{\frac{n}{2}} \exp\left\{-\sum_{i=1}^{n} \frac{(y_i - \mu)^2}{2}\right\} \\
&= \left(\frac{1}{2\pi}\right)^{\frac{n}{2}} \exp\left\{-\sum_{i=1}^{n} \frac{y_i^2}{2}\right\} \exp\left\{\mu T(y) - \frac{n\mu^2}{2}\right\} \\
&= c(y) L^*(\mu; T(y)).
\end{aligned}
$$

Thus, all of our inferences about the mean cholesterol level μ can be based on the likelihood function L^*, which depends only on the sample through the value of the sum of all cholesterol levels in the sample. That is, the sum of all cholesterol levels is a sufficient statistic and the sample can be reduced to this statistic without losing any information. Notice that the obvious estimate of μ, the sample mean, is indeed able to be calculated based on this sufficient statistic. Of course, it is important to remember that we have assumed the population variance cholesterol level is known. If this were not the case, and we wanted to simultaneously assess the support for values of σ^2, then the above conclusion is not true as we will see in Example 3.5.

The concept of sufficiency allows us to judge whether a particular statistic contains all the available information in the sample. However, it does not tell us which sufficient statistic is most concise, or achieves the most data reduction. For example, the full sample $y = (y_1, \ldots, y_n)$ is always a sufficient statistic, but if the sample sum $\sum y_i$ is also a sufficient statistic then we would prefer to use the sum since it is more concise. This highlights the fact that we generally prefer a **minimal sufficient statistic**. Intuitively, this means a sufficient statistic that most concisely conveys the information available in the sample. More precisely, a sufficient statistic is called a minimal sufficient statistic if it can be written as a function of any other sufficient statistic. This means that the extent of data reduction is greatest with a minimal sufficient statistic.

Minimal sufficient statistics can be identified using a mathematical criterion that follows from the factorisation criterion for sufficiency. In particular, a sufficient statistic $T(y)$ is a minimal sufficient statistic if, for any two values of the sample y_1 and y_2,

$$
\frac{L(\theta; y_1)}{L(\theta; y_2)} \text{ is independent of } \theta \text{ if and only if } T(y_1) = T(y_2).
$$

While this criterion can be useful for determining whether a sufficient statistic is also minimal sufficient, it is worth noting that for many commonly used parametric models the sufficient statistic that arises naturally from the factorisation criterion is also a minimal sufficient statistic. For example, in Example 3.4 the sufficient statistic $T(y) = \sum_{i=1}^{n} y_i$ is also a minimal sufficient statistic, as will be verified in the exercises.

3.5 Multiple parameters

Our discussion and examples of the likelihood function have generally been framed in terms of a single parameter. However, everything that we have discussed so far is also appropriate when θ is a vector $\theta = (\theta_1, \ldots, \theta_p)$. In this case the likelihood function is a function of several variables, and it measures the support that the data provide for the entire combination of values of the several parameters. When there are just two parameters, it is still possible to plot the likelihood function using 3-dimensional graphics; however, for three or more parameters it is of course not possible to display the complete likelihood function graphically. Nonetheless, our definition and interpretation of the likelihood and log-likelihood functions are still relevant when there are multiple parameters. Our definitions of a sufficient statistic and a minimal sufficient statistic also remain the same, although in this case it will often be the case that such statistics are vectors, as is illustrated in the following example.

Example 3.5 Now consider our cholesterol level study again, but without the assumption that we know what the population variance cholesterol level is. The likelihood function is therefore a function of two parameters

$$L(\mu, \sigma^2) = \left(\frac{1}{2\pi\sigma^2}\right)^{\frac{n}{2}} \exp\left\{-\sum_{i=1}^{n} \frac{(y_i - \mu)^2}{2\sigma^2}\right\}.$$

The value of the likelihood function for a particular combination of values for μ and σ^2 measures the support the data has for that combination of parameter values. Thus, for example, if the likelihood associated with the values $\mu = 5.1$ and $\sigma^2 = 0.7$ is greater than the likelihood associated with the values $\mu = 5.9$ and $\sigma^2 = 4.5$, then this means that the former combination of parameter values is more supported than the latter combination. Note that we have not split up the support for values of μ from the support for values of σ^2. Rather, the likelihood measures the support for a particular combination of parameter values. Now consider the following statistic, which is a vector,

$$T(y) = (T_1(y), T_2(y)) = \left(\sum_{i=1}^{n} y_i, \sum_{i=1}^{n} y_i^2\right).$$

Then the likelihood function can written as

$$
\begin{aligned}
L(\mu, \sigma^2) &= \left(\frac{1}{2\pi\sigma^2}\right)^{\frac{n}{2}} \exp\left\{-\frac{1}{2\sigma^2}\left(T_2(y) - 2\mu T_1(y) + n\mu^2\right)\right\} \\
&= c(y)L^*(\mu, \sigma^2; T(y)).
\end{aligned}
$$

Thus, collectively, the sum of the cholesterol levels and the sum of the squared cholesterol levels are sufficient to convey all the available information in the sample about the population mean and variance. Note that the obvious estimates of μ and σ^2, the sample mean and variance, are able to be calculated based on these two statistics.

3.6 Nuisance parameters

When the likelihood function is a function of several parameters, then it is sometimes the case that not all of the parameters are of equal interest. Indeed, in some instances one or more of the parameters may be of no interest at all. In this case, the presence of these parameters in our likelihood function is a nuisance, as it will complicate any analyses that we conduct based on the likelihood function. Such parameters are referred to as **nuisance parameters**, and we may try to simplify our likelihood function by eliminating these parameters, thus allowing us to focus on the parameters that we are interested in.

There are a few approaches that we can take to simplify our likelihood so that it no longer depends on the nuisance parameters. Here we will focus on just one approach, which is an approach that is always applicable in principle, and which is based on the fairly obvious idea of getting rid of the nuisance parameters by replacing them with estimates. When we replace the nuisance parameters with estimates in the likelihood function, then the resulting function only depends on the parameters of interest, and is referred to as a **profile likelihood**. The profile likelihood can then be used to obtain information about the parameters of interest. While this approach may seem fairly straightforward, in practice there are a number of complications that must be considered, such as how we estimate the nuisance parameters to construct the profile likelihood.

Suppose we have two parameters in our parametric model, θ and β, and suppose that we are interested only in θ. Then our approach is to replace the nuisance parameter β by an estimate, $\hat{\beta}$, in the likelihood function $L(\theta, \beta)$. By substituting this estimate into the likelihood function, the resulting function depends only on θ, $L(\theta) = L(\theta, \hat{\beta})$, and it is $L(\theta)$ that we refer to as the profile likelihood. The profile likelihood can be used to measure the support that the data provide for any given value of θ and it is simpler than the real likelihood function in the sense that it does not depend on the nuisance parameter β.

A straightforward example would be the case where we are interested only in the mean cholesterol level based on our previous normal distribution model, and the unknown variance of the cholesterol level in our model is a nuisance. Then instead of the full likelihood we discussed in Example 3.5, we could measure support for different values of the mean μ using the profile likelihood $L(\mu) = L(\mu, s^2)$. This is a function only of μ, once we have calculated and substituted in the value of the sample variance s^2.

The normal distribution example is particularly simple by virtue of the fact that the sample variance s^2 is a sensible estimate of σ^2 regardless of the value that μ takes. This means that we only have to estimate $\beta = \sigma^2$ once and substitute it into the likelihood function to obtain the profile likelihood as a function of $\theta = \mu$. For other models this may not always be the case, because there may be no single estimate of β that makes sense regardless of the value of θ. In such cases a different estimate of β would be required for each different value of θ. That is, we would need to consider our estimate of β to be a function of θ, $\hat{\beta}(\theta)$, and then the profile likelihood for θ becomes

$$L(\theta) = L(\theta, \hat{\beta}(\theta)).$$

Notice that θ now occurs in two places in the profile likelihood. Nonetheless, the resulting profile likelihood is a function of θ alone and can be used to measure the support for specific values of θ, independently of β.

Of course, there remains the question of how to choose the estimate for β. In general, for a given value of θ, the estimate of β is always the value that is most supported by the data. In other words, for each possible value of θ, $\hat{\beta}(\theta)$ is the value of β that achieves the greatest likelihood value. The idea of using an estimate that corresponds to the value that is most supported by the data is a key concept in statistical inference, and we will return to this idea in some detail when we discuss maximum likelihood estimation in Chapter 4. In this chapter, however, we focus our discussion on illustrating the construction of profile likelihoods when the estimate of β depends on θ, as presented in Section 3.7.5 of the extended example.

Finally, we note that profile likelihood is not the only way that a nuisance parameter can be eliminated from the likelihood function. Various other types of modified likelihood functions exist that allow an assessment of the level of support for specific values of the parameter of interest, independently of the nuisance parameter. Some commonly used approaches that are useful in specific applications include **conditional likelihood**, **marginal likelihood** and **partial likelihood**. Like the profile likelihood, these approaches all involve reducing the full likelihood function to a function that involves just the parameters of interest, and then using this function in the same way as a likelihood function. A detailed study of these modified likelihood functions is beyond our scope, but a good starting point for further reading is the chapter on modified likelihoods in the book by Cox (2006).

3.7 Extended example

In this extended example we consider the construction of likelihood functions associated with disease incidence rates, using a parametric model based on the Poisson distribution. We begin by discussing the likelihood function for a single incidence rate. The objective is to illustrate the use of the likelihood function for comparing different values of the disease incidence rate with respect to their support from the data, as well as to illustrate the notion of data reduction and sufficiency. We then extend the discussion to likelihood functions relating to two incidence rates, and in particular how to create a likelihood function for the incidence rate ratio, which is of interest in comparing the rate of disease in two populations. In addition to illustrating likelihood functions for multiple parameters, the rate ratio context also provides an example where nuisance parameters arise, and allows us to consider ways in which nuisance parameters can be eliminated from likelihood functions.

3.7.1 Modelling stroke incidence

Disease incidence is typically studied in the context of epidemiological cohort studies, where individuals are followed prospectively over time for the occurrence of new cases of a particular disease. Often one of the primary aims is to compare two exposure groups with respect to the rate at which disease occurs, in the hope that conclusions can be made about the association between exposure and disease. In this extended example we will consider the example of stroke incidence among people who have a past history of coronary disease, and suppose that we have been able to follow two such groups of patients, one group exposed to a high salt diet (group 1) and the other to a low salt diet (group 2). We will suppose that during the period of follow-up, we observe Y_1 new cases of stroke in the high salt group, and Y_2 new cases of stroke in the low salt group. These strokes were observed among $n_1 = 1150$ individuals in the low salt group and $n_2 = 850$ individuals in the high salt group. The average length of follow-up for each individual was 5.2 years in the low salt group, and 4.5 years in the high salt group, or equivalently, a total follow-up of $F_1 = 5.2 \times 1150 = 5980$ person-years and $F_2 = 4.5 \times 850 = 3825$ person-years, respectively. Our goal is to obtain information about the rate at which new cases of stroke occur per person per year, in the population from which these individuals were taken.

Let λ_1 and λ_2 be the rates of new stroke cases in the population of individuals that follow low salt diets and high salt diets, respectively. Remember that λ_1 and λ_2 are the true rates in the population, which must be carefully distinguished from the observed rates in our hypothetical study. As always, it is the task of statistical inference to quantify the extent to which the observed (sample) values give us reliable information about the true (population) values. If the true rate of strokes in the low salt population were 0.0063 per year, this would mean, for example, that if we followed a group of individuals having a low salt diet, for a total of 1200 person years, we would expect on average to observe $1200 \times 0.0063 = 7.56$ new strokes. More generally, the expected number of strokes in group i is $\lambda_i F_i$, and the distribution of the number of strokes can be modelled using a Poisson$(\lambda_i F_i)$ distribution,

$$f_i(y_i; \lambda_i) = \Pr(Y_i = y_i) = \frac{(\lambda_i F_i)^{y_i} \exp(-\lambda_i F_i)}{y_i!}.$$

An important assumption is that we consider the lengths of follow-up, F_i, to be fixed constants in much the same way as the sample size in a disease prevalence study was considered fixed in Chapter 1. This leads to a parametric model for our sample $Y = (Y_1, Y_2)$, and in the next section we shall consider the likelihood function corresponding to this parametric model, under the initial assumption that the incidence rates in the two groups are equal. In subsequent sections, this assumption will be relaxed. Note that the Poisson model is a popular parametric model for disease incidence counts, however, it is not the only model that could be used. An important assumption in what is to follow is that the Poisson model is an appropriate model for the way the data arose. Usually this will be the case when individuals in the study are independent of each other. You might like to think about ways in which this assumption could possibly be violated in the present context, although we shall not consider alternative models here.

3.7.2 Likelihood function for a common rate

To begin with we will assume that there is no difference between the two dietary groups with respect to stroke rates, and discuss the likelihood function for the common incidence rate $\lambda = \lambda_1 = \lambda_2$. A reasonable assumption for this study is that the two dietary groups behave independently, in which case the joint probability function for the sample $Y = (Y_1, Y_2)$ is the product of the individual probability functions,

$$f_Y(y; \lambda) = f_1(y_1; \lambda) f_2(y_2; \lambda) = \frac{F_1^{y_1} F_2^{y_2} \lambda^{y_1 + y_2} \exp\{-\lambda(F_1 + F_2)\}}{y_1! y_2!}.$$

Suppose we observe a particular sample of stroke counts, say

$$y = (y_1, y_2) = (245, 239).$$

For any given value of the population incidence rate, say λ_0, the likelihood of that value may be interpreted as the probability that we would have observed 245 strokes among individuals on a low salt diet and 239 strokes among individuals on a high salt diet, if the true value of λ is λ_0. Thus, considering all the possible values of $\lambda > 0$, the likelihood function for λ is therefore the above probability function, considered as a function of λ instead of y. Substituting in the fixed constant values of F_1 and F_2 from the previous section, and letting

$$c(y) = \frac{F_1^{y_1} F_2^{y_2}}{y_1! y_2!} = \frac{5980^{y_1} 3825^{y_2}}{y_1! y_2!}$$

leads to the following likelihood function for the incidence rate:

$$L(\lambda) = L(\lambda;y) = c(y)\lambda^{y_1+y_2}\exp(-9805\lambda).$$

The corresponding log-likelihood function is

$$\ell(\lambda) = \log L(\lambda) = \log c(y) + (y_1+y_2)\log\lambda - 9805\lambda.$$

The likelihood (and log-likelihood) allows us to compare different possible values of the population stroke incidence rate, in terms of the extent to which the data support such values. Consider, for example, the following two possible estimates of the stroke rate, per person per year:

$$\frac{y_1+y_2}{F_1+F_2} = \frac{245+239}{5980+3825} = 0.0494$$

and

$$\frac{1}{2}\left(\frac{y_1}{F_1}+\frac{y_2}{F_2}\right) = \frac{1}{2}\left(\frac{245}{5980}+\frac{239}{3825}\right) = 0.0517.$$

Notice that the first estimate is the total number of strokes in the two groups divided by the total person-years of follow-up, while the second estimate is the average of the incidence rate estimates from the two groups. The likelihood values corresponding to these two parameter values are $L(0.0494) = 1.514 \times 10^{-8}$ and $L(0.0517) = 0.884 \times 10^{-8}$, with a likelihood ratio of 1.71. Equivalently, the log-likelihood values corresponding to these two parameter values are $\ell(0.0494) = -18.0058$ and $\ell(0.0517) = -18.5438$, with a log-likelihood difference of 0.538. The absolute likelihood values are exceedingly small but they have little meaning on their own. It is their relative magnitudes, as indicated by the likelihood ratio and log-likelihood difference, that are useful for comparative purposes. It can be seen that the likelihood ratio (or equivalently the log-likelihood difference) indicates that the value 0.0494 is more supported by the data than the value 0.0517.

We can consider more fully the support provided for different values of the parameter, by looking at the entire likelihood and log-likelihood functions. A plot of the likelihood function is provided in Figure 3.3, together with the values of the two potential estimates of λ. As well as illustrating better support for the value 0.0494, notice that this value is the most supported value, in the sense that it achieves the highest likelihood of any value. This is not a coincidence, and we return in Chapter 4 to the use of this criterion for estimating parameters, including the construction of confidence intervals.

3.7.3 Data reduction

If the population stroke rates for the two diets are identical, then intuitively it would seem that there is nothing to be gained by collecting our data broken up into the two groups. We can confirm this using the concept of a sufficient statistic. Notice first of all that the likelihood function described in the previous section can be written as

$$L(\lambda) = L(\lambda;y) = c(y)L^*(\lambda;y)$$

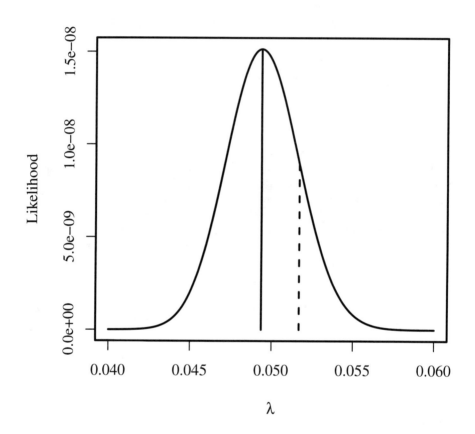

FIGURE 3.3
Likelihood function for the common stroke rate λ, with the values 0.0494 (solid line) and 0.0517 (dashed line) identified

where

$$L^*(\lambda;y) = \lambda^{y_1 + y_2} \exp(-9805\lambda).$$

As discussed earlier in this chapter, since the term $c(y)$ does not depend on the parameter λ we can use $L^*(\lambda;y)$ as the likelihood function, and this would lead to exactly the same likelihood ratios (and log-likelihood differences) for comparing the support for different potential incidence rate values. Of primary importance is the fact that $L^*(\lambda;y)$ only depends on the sample through the observed value of the statistic $T(y) = y_1 + y_2$. It follows that the total number of stroke cases is all that is required to obtain information about the incidence rate when using the likelihood function. That is, the total number of stroke cases is a sufficient statistic, and breaking the number of cases down into the two groups does not provide any extra information about the stroke incidence rate. This is consistent with the fact that in the previous section, the better supported estimate of λ was able to be calculated using only knowledge of the total number of strokes, whereas the lesser supported estimate used the number of strokes in each dietary group.

3.7.4   Likelihood function for the rate ratio

Suppose now that we are not prepared to make the assumption that the two diets are associated with the same stroke incidence rate, and indeed are interested in assessing the degree to which the data support (or do not support) identical stroke rates. Going back to the joint probability function without the assumption $\lambda = \lambda_1 = \lambda_2$, and dropping factors that do not depend on the parameters λ_1 or λ_2, leads to the following likelihood and log-likelihood functions:

$$L(\lambda_1, \lambda_2) = \lambda_1^{y_1} \lambda_2^{y_2} \exp(-5980\lambda_1 - 3825\lambda_2)$$

and

$$\ell(\lambda_1, \lambda_2) = y_1 \log(\lambda_1) + y_2 \log(\lambda_2) - 5980\lambda_1 - 3825\lambda_2.$$

In epidemiology, a standard way to measure the relative sizes of two incidence rates is via the rate ratio, which we will denote by $\gamma = \lambda_2/\lambda_1$. When this rate ratio is 1 then the incidence rate is equal in the two groups, and values different from 1 indicate unequal incidence rates. For the purpose of assessing the support for different values of the rate ratio, it would be more convenient if our likelihood function were a function of γ. By using the relationship $\lambda_1 = \gamma\lambda_2$, we can rewrite the likelihood function as a function of λ_1 and γ. This leads to the following likelihood and log-likelihood functions, substituting in the observed sample values $y = (y_1, y_2) = (245, 239)$:

$$L(\lambda_1, \gamma) = \lambda_1^{245} (\gamma\lambda_1)^{239} \exp(-5980\lambda_1 - 3825\gamma\lambda_1)$$

and

$$\ell(\lambda_1, \gamma) = 245 \log(\lambda_1) + 239 \log(\gamma\lambda_1) - 5980\lambda_1 - 3825\gamma\lambda_1.$$

This rewriting of the likelihood function is an example of a technique called **reparameterisation**. It means that we can now explicitly assess the support for different values of the rate ratio (concurrently with values of the incidence rate in the low salt diet population).

Because we now have two parameters, the likelihood function is a function of two variables. Therefore, in studying the support for different values of the rate ratio, we need to concurrently specify the value of the other parameter λ_1. The sample incidence rates in the two groups, as used in the exercises of Chapter 1, provide estimates of the stroke rates in each group,

$$\hat{\lambda}_1 = \frac{245}{5980} = 0.0410 \qquad \text{and} \qquad \hat{\lambda}_2 = \frac{239}{3825} = 0.0625$$

and suggest a possible estimate of the rate ratio $\hat{\gamma} = 0.0625/0.0410 = 1.52$. Consider the extent to which the sample supports the parameter combination $(\lambda_1, \gamma) = (0.0410, 1.52)$, compared to the parameter combination $(\lambda_1, \gamma) = (0.0410, 1)$. This comparison effectively allows us to compare the relative support for equal versus unequal stroke rates, assuming the low salt diet stroke rate is 0.0410. The likelihood ratio corresponding to these two combinations is

$$\frac{L(0.0410, 1.52)}{L(0.0410, 1)} = 1.11 \times 10^8.$$

This value indicates that if the low salt stroke rate is 0.0410 per person per year, then the data provide more support for unequal stroke rates than for equal stroke rates. Indeed, the magnitude of the likelihood ratio seems to indicate that there is substantially more support. (In Chapter 6 we shall discuss how to interpret more formally the magnitude of the likelihood ratio for the purpose of assessing whether there is "significant" evidence against the hypothesis of equal stroke rates.) We might also consider a comparison of the support for these two rate ratio values in conjunction with a different value for λ_1. For example, the likelihood values for the two combinations $(\lambda_1, \gamma) = (0.05, 1.52)$ and $(\lambda_1, \gamma) = (0.05, 1)$ lead to a likelihood ratio of 1.86, which again suggests greater support for a rate ratio value that is different from 1.

While our two likelihood comparisons above were consistent in that they both indicated greater support for the parameter combination with rate ratio greater than 1, notice that the actual magnitude of the likelihood ratio was dramatically different in the two comparisons. That is, the magnitude of the likelihood ratio depends on the value chosen for λ_1. If our primary interest is in comparison of the stroke rates in the two groups, in other words in the rate ratio, then it is a nuisance that we need to specify the value of λ_1 in order to compare the support for different values of the rate ratio γ. In the terminology used earlier in this chapter, λ_1 is a nuisance parameter. Next we discuss how to eliminate the nuisance parameter from the likelihood function so that we can compare the support for different values of the rate ratio without having to specify the value of the nuisance parameter.

3.7.5   Eliminating the nuisance parameter

In Section 3.6 we discussed the idea of eliminating a nuisance parameter by using a profile likelihood, which involves using an estimate of the nuisance parameter. We

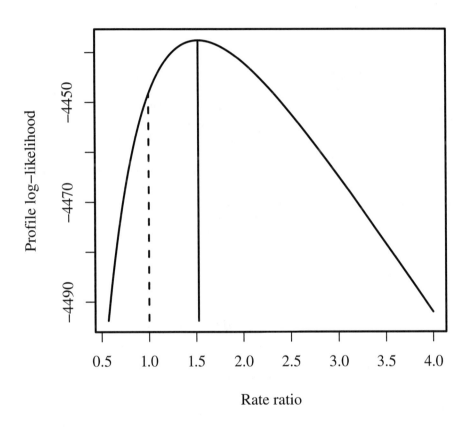

FIGURE 3.4
Profile log-likelihood function for the rate ratio, with the values 1 (dashed line) and 1.52 (solid line) identified

now consider this approach in order to eliminate λ_1 from the likelihood function. In the present context, for any value of γ for which we would like to assess the level of support, we need to substitute into the likelihood function an estimate of λ_1. Having substituted in the estimate of λ_1, the likelihood will depend only on γ, and we will be able to evaluate the likelihood at the particular value of γ that we are interested in. The question remains: what estimate of λ_1 should we substitute into the likelihood? The best estimate of λ_1 will depend on the particular value of γ that we are interested in calculating the likelihood for. It turns out that if we assume a particular value of γ then the most supported value of λ_1 is

$$\hat{\lambda}_1(\gamma) = \frac{y_1 + y_2}{F_1 + \gamma F_2}.$$

We will return to why this is the case in Chapter 4, when we discuss the use of the most supported value as an estimate. For now, we will take it as a given that $\hat{\lambda}_1(\gamma)$ is an appropriate estimate of λ_1 assuming a particular value for γ. Substituting our estimate of λ_1 into our likelihood function, in other words replacing λ_1 by $\hat{\lambda}_1(\gamma)$ in the likelihood function, leads to a function that depends only on γ. We refer to this function as a profile likelihood function, and it allows us to assess and compare the level of support for different values of the stroke rate ratio, without the nuisance of having to concurrently specify a value for the stroke rate in the low salt group. Making the necessary substitutions into the likelihood function, and dropping any factors that do not depend on the remaining parameter γ, leads to the following profile likelihood and log-likelihood functions for our sample:

$$L(\gamma) = \frac{\gamma^{239}}{(5980 + 3825\gamma)^{484}}$$

and

$$\ell(\gamma) = 239\log(\gamma) - 484\log(5980 + 3825\gamma).$$

Recall that in the previous section we were interested in comparing the level of support for the two rate ratio values 1.52 and 1. Using the profile likelihood we can do this without the nuisance of having to specify which value of λ_1 we are assuming. Figure 3.4 provides a plot of the profile log-likelihood function for our sample. It can be seen that the value 1.52, corresponding to a higher stroke rate in the high salt group, has greater support from the data than the value 1, corresponding to equal stroke rates. Whether the amount of additional support is "statistically significant" is something that we will leave until we discuss hypothesis testing in Chapter 6. However, if it were, then this would indicate an association between salt intake and stroke rates. Of course, since this is an epidemiological study in which individuals choose their own diet, rather than a randomised study in which they are randomly assigned their diet, the cause of the apparent association is not clear. It could be because higher salt intake leads to a higher risk of stroke, or it could be because people who happen to have a high salt intake tend to have other characteristics that make them more prone to stroke.

Exercises

1. In a study of late stage terminal cancer, the time from disease progression until death was observed in a random sample of $n = 100$ patients, giving the observed sample $y_1, \ldots, y_{100}$. The sample mean was $\bar{y} = 3.2$ months and the sample median was $m = 2.7$ months. The exponential distribution with parameter λ and probability density function

$$f_i(y_i; \lambda) = \lambda e^{-\lambda y_i} \qquad \lambda > 0$$

is a common parametric model for observations that involve observing the time until an event occurs. The parameter λ can be interpreted as the rate of death per person per month. Since the expectation and median of the exponential distribution are $1/\lambda$ and $\log(2)/\lambda$, respectively, the following are both natural estimates of λ

$$\hat{\lambda}_1 = \frac{1}{\bar{y}} \qquad \hat{\lambda}_2 = \frac{\log(2)}{m}.$$

   (a) Write down the likelihood function and the log-likelihood function for the death rate λ.

   (b) Use the factorisation criterion to find a sufficient statistic for λ. Is this statistic minimal sufficient?

   (c) For the sample described above, which of the two estimates, $\hat{\lambda}_1$ or $\hat{\lambda}_2$, is more supported by the data.

   (d) Show that the result obtained in part (c) is in fact true for all samples, not just the one described above.

   (e) Comment on the results of parts (b) and (d).

2. Consider the observed value of an independent random sample $y = (y_1, \ldots, y_n)$ taken from a $N(\mu, 1)$ distribution. In Example 3.4 we demonstrated that

$$T(y) = \sum_{i=1}^{n} y_i$$

is a sufficient statistic for μ. Show that $T(y)$ is a minimal sufficient statistic for μ.

3. A study was conducted to investigate the variability of a laboratory assay used to measure HIV viral load, the concentration of virus in the blood. For each of n HIV infected people, two blood samples were taken one day apart, and the viral load was measured using each sample. Since the underlying "true" viral load would not be expected to have changed during one day, any differences between the measurements in the two blood samples may be attributed to assay variability. If we let d_i be the observed difference between the first and second

measurement for individual i, then a common model would be to assume that d_i is the observed value of a random variable $D_i \overset{d}{=} N(0, \sigma^2)$. The variance of this distribution, $\sigma^2 = \mathrm{Var}(D_i)$, provides information about the assay variability.

(a) Write down the likelihood function and the log-likelihood function for the variance σ^2.

(b) Use the factorisation criterion to find a sufficient statistic for σ^2. Is this statistic minimal sufficient?

(c) Either version of the sample variance of the d_i values, s_n^2 or s_{n-1}^2, is a possible estimate of σ^2. Show that these estimates cannot be calculated using only the observed value of the sufficient statistic from part (b).

(d) Explain why no information has been lost by reducing the sample down to the sufficient statistic, even though the sample variance can no longer be calculated.

(e) Suggest another estimate of σ^2, s_d^2, that can be calculated using only the observed value of the sufficient statistic.

(f) In a sample of $n = 5$ HIV infected people, the differences between their two viral load measurements were

$$d_1 = -0.7 \qquad d_2 = 0.5 \qquad d_3 = 0.1 \qquad d_4 = 1.0 \qquad d_5 = -0.1.$$

Which of the three estimates, s_n^2, s_{n-1}^2 or s_d^2, is most supported by the data?

4. Consider the following study of fertility, and its association with smoking exposure. We take a random sample of n mothers giving birth for the first time, n_1 of whom are non-smokers and n_2 of whom are smokers, where $n_1 + n_2 = n$. At the time of giving birth we collect information on the number of attempts (conception cycles) required to achieve the pregnancy. For mothers in the first group we will let the number of attempts be x_i, $i = 1, \ldots, n_1$, and for mothers in the second group we will let the number of attempts be y_i, $i = 1, \ldots, n_2$. We will model the number of attempts using a geometric distribution, with separate distributions in the two groups. In group 1 (non-smokers), the number of attempts for woman i will have the following probability function

$$f(x_i; p_1) = \Pr(X_i = x_i) = p_1(1 - p_1)^{x_i - 1}$$

where $x_i = 1, 2, \ldots$ and $0 < p_1 \leq 1$. In group 2 (smokers), the number of attempts for woman i will have the following probability function

$$f(y_i; p_2) = \Pr(Y_i = y_i) = p_2(1 - p_2)^{y_i - 1}$$

where $y_i = 1, 2, \ldots$ and $0 < p_2 \leq 1$.

(a) Review the definition of the geometric distribution. Why does the geometric distribution provide a natural probability model for this study?

(b) What is the interpretation of the parameters p_1 and p_2 in the above fertility model?

(c) What is the interpretation of $\gamma = p_1/p_2$?

5. Suppose that the study in Exercise 4 had only collected information on mothers who are non-smokers. Write down the likelihood function and the log-likelihood function for p_1, based on the sample $(x_1, \ldots, x_{n_1})$.

6. Now consider the full sample from Exercise 4, $(x_1, \ldots, x_{n_1})$ and $(y_1, \ldots, y_{n_2})$, but suppose that the fertility parameters in the two groups are identical, $p = p_1 = p_2$.

    (a) Write down the likelihood and log-likelihood functions for p, based on the sample $(x_1, \ldots, x_{n_1}, y_1, \ldots, y_{n_2})$.

    (b) By finding a sufficient statistic, justify that all the information in this sample concerning p is contained in a single number, the total number of pregnancy attempts by all women from both groups.

7. Under the assumptions of Exercise 6, consider a particular study in which we observe $n_1 = 78$ mothers who are non-smokers and $n_2 = 51$ mothers who are smokers. The mothers in group 1 had a total of $\sum x_i = 207$ pregnancy attempts, and the mothers in group 2 had a total of $\sum y_i = 212$ pregnancy attempts.

    (a) Substitute the above sample values into the likelihood function from Exercise 6, and hence plot the likelihood function for p.

    (b) Calculate the following two possible estimates of p

    $$\frac{n_1 + n_2}{\sum x_i + \sum y_i} \quad \text{and} \quad \frac{1}{2}\left(\frac{n_1}{\sum x_i} + \frac{n_2}{\sum y_i}\right).$$

    (c) Calculate the likelihood ratio and log-likelihood difference for comparing the support for each of these possible values of p. Which estimate is better supported by the data?

    (d) Mark both estimates on your plot of the likelihood function from part (a). Does there seem to be a better supported value than either of these?

8. Suppose now that we are not prepared to assume that the fertility parameters are the same in the two groups, and that we want to compare the fertility using the relative fertility rate γ.

    (a) Using the sample described in Exercise 7, write down the likelihood and log-likelihood functions for p_1 and p_2, that is, $L(p_1, p_2)$ and $\ell(p_1, p_2)$.

    (b) Using the relationship $p_1 = p_2\gamma$, rewrite the likelihood function and log-likelihood functions in terms of p_2 and γ, that is, $L(\gamma, p_2)$ and $\ell(\gamma, p_2)$.

(c) A possible estimate of γ is $\bar{y}/\bar{x} = 1.57$. Suppose we want to compare whether this value is better supported by the data than the value 1 (the value 1 would indicate no difference in the fertility of mothers from the two groups). Calculate the likelihood ratio comparing these two values, firstly assuming $p_2 = 0.25$ and secondly assuming $p_2 = 0.50$. Does the result depend on the value of p_2 that we assume?

(d) Suppose you are told that for any given value of γ, the best estimate of p_2 is

$$\hat{p}_2(\gamma) = \frac{1}{\bar{x}\gamma} = \frac{0.377}{\gamma}.$$

Substitute $\hat{p}_2(\gamma)$ into the log-likelihood in place of p_2 to end up with a function of γ only. Plot this function, which is called the profile log-likelihood function.

(e) Using the plot in part (d), what is the most supported value for γ, based on the profile log-likelihood? What is the interpretation of this value in terms of the relative fertility of the two groups of mothers?

4

Estimation methods

The likelihood function discussed in Chapter 3 allows us to compare two parameter values with respect to the level of support that the sample provides for these values, and hence to decide whether one parameter value has more support than another. The objective of this chapter is to use the concept of likelihood to motivate a general method of estimation, by identifying the most supported value out of all possible values of the parameter. This is referred to as maximum likelihood estimation, and can be used to provide estimates in situations where there is no obvious way to estimate the parameter. We begin by discussing how to define the maximum likelihood estimator followed by a discussion of the concept of statistical information, and its use in providing standard errors and confidence intervals associated with maximum likelihood estimates. We then consider properties of maximum likelihood estimation, using the estimation concepts discussed in Chapter 2, and will see that it generally provides the best possible approach to estimation. While maximum likelihood estimation is the most important general approach, we will also discuss some alternative methods that are useful in specific contexts, particularly the method of least squares estimation. We then illustrate the concepts by continuing our disease incidence example from Chapter 3.

4.1 Maximum likelihood estimation

Consider an observed sample $y = (y_1 \ldots, y_n)$ and likelihood function $L(\theta) = L(\theta;y)$. Recall that the likelihood associated with a particular parameter value θ_0 is the probability (density) of obtaining the sample y, assuming that the true value of the parameter is θ_0. This measures the support that the data has for the parameter value θ_0, and the most supported parameter value $\hat{\theta}$ will be the value for which $L(\hat{\theta}) > L(\theta_0)$ whenever $\theta_0 \neq \hat{\theta}$. The most supported parameter value is therefore the value that achieves the highest likelihood possible based on the likelihood function $L(\theta)$, or in other words maximises the likelihood function. Since this value has more support from the data than any other parameter value it makes sense to use it as our estimate. This approach to estimation is referred to as **maximum likelihood estimation** and can be interpreted as providing the parameter value that makes the observed sample the most likely sample among all possible samples. The estimate that arises from using this approach, which will be a function of the observed sample $\hat{\theta} = \Theta(y)$, is referred to as the **maximum likelihood estimate**. As with any estimate, it is the observed value of a random variable, the **maximum likelihood estimator** $\hat{\Theta} = \Theta(Y)$. The abbreviation **MLE** is used interchangeably to refer to both the maximum likelihood estimate or the maximum likelihood estimator, depending on the context.

Maximum likelihood estimation provides a general approach to estimating a parameter, and can in principle be applied in any situation where we have a likelihood function. In our discussions about estimation in Chapter 2, we relied on being able to choose estimates that made intuitive sense based on the situation under study. For example, we used the sample mean to estimate the population mean, and the sample variance to estimate the population variance. In more complicated situations, it is usually not possible to find an intuitively natural estimate such as the sample mean or variance, and the principle of maximum likelihood estimation provides a generally applicable criterion on which to base our parameter estimate.

While it is straightforward to define the MLE as the parameter value that achieves the highest likelihood, there are a number of potentially important details that we need to be aware of. The discussion above is framed as though there could only ever be one value of the parameter that maximises the likelihood function. While it is often the case that there is only one unique maximum for the likelihood function, it is possible in complicated situations for there to be two or more values of the parameter that achieve the highest possible value for the likelihood function. In such situations we say that the MLE is not unique, and it may not be clear which parameter value to use as our estimate. While this is a cause for concern when it arises, it turns out that in most contexts of interest the MLE is unique and this potential complication does not arise. Another important detail in relation to our definition of the MLE is our choice of the parameter space, that is, the set of all possible values that the parameter can have. When finding the MLE we must consider only those values of the parameter that are within the parameter space, even though the function $L(\theta)$ may be evaluable for values of θ that are not in the parameter space. For example, if our parameter is a proportion such as the population prevalence of disease, then we must restrict our attention to the range of parameter values between 0 and 1 when finding the prevalence value that has the highest likelihood. This could be an important point if the likelihood function is able to take on larger values when the prevalence is outside the interval 0 to 1, than when it is inside this interval.

Bearing in mind these potential complexities, an MLE is strictly speaking defined as any value $\hat{\theta}$ that is in the parameter space and for which $L(\hat{\theta}) \geq L(\theta_0)$ for any other parameter value θ_0 that is also in the parameter space. In mathematical parlance, we say that the MLE is the value that maximises $L(\theta)$ over the parameter space. In practice, however, this often simply amounts to taking the MLE to be the single value of θ that leads to function $L(\theta)$ taking on its highest possible value.

As a final point of importance in defining the MLE, recall from the discussion in Chapter 3 that if a particular parameter value maximises the likelihood function then it will also maximise the log-likelihood function. Thus, the above definition of the MLE can also be made with respect to the log-likelihood function $\ell(\theta)$ rather than the likelihood $L(\theta)$. In practice, this fact is often used for computation purposes because the log-likelihood function is usually a more mathematically convenient function to deal with.

Example 4.1 In Chapter 3 we studied the likelihood function associated with a fertility study in which the sample corresponds to the number of conception cycles until pregnancy, y_i, for a sample of n couples having their first child. Throughout this chapter we will use this as an example of maximum likelihood estimation, restricting ourselves to the simpler situation where there is no difference in the fertility of mothers exposed to smoking compared those not exposed. Recall that for this situation a sufficient statistic is the total number of pregnancy attempts by all couples, $y = \sum_i y_i$, and the likelihood function based on the geometric distribution can be written as

$$L(p) = p^n(1-p)^{y-n}$$

where the parameter p is the probability of success for a single cycle. The parameter space in this model is the interval $(0,1]$ so the MLE is defined as the maximum of the likelihood function over the interval $(0,1]$. Note, however, that it is possible to evaluate the function $L(p)$ for values of p outside this interval, and these values must be ignored in determining the MLE. Consider a sample in which $n = 2$ couples take a total of $y = 4$ attempts to achieve their first pregnancy. Figure 4.1 plots the likelihood function

$$L(p) = p^2(1-p)^2$$

over the parameter space and outside the parameter space, together with the MLE as the maximum of the likelihood over the parameter space. It is seen that the maximum of the likelihood function over the parameter space occurs at the MLE $\hat{p} = 0.5$, corresponding to an estimated 50% probability of pregnancy in any given cycle. Notice that $L(p)$ may achieve higher values outside the parameter space, however, these are of no relevance for determining the MLE.

4.2 Calculation of the MLE

Our discussion in this section and most of this chapter will be framed in terms of estimation of a single parameter, however, we will provide a discussion of the multiple parameter situation at the end of the chapter, where it will be seen that many of the concepts discussed carry over quite naturally.

Calculation of an MLE requires us to maximise a function. Very commonly, although not necessarily always, calculus is a useful tool for carrying out this maximisation. In many contexts, the maximum value of the likelihood function, or equivalently the log-likelihood function, occurs at a stationary point where the derivative is zero. Under these circumstances the MLE can be found by solving an equation that involves setting the derivative of the log-likelihood function, with respect to the parameter θ, equal to zero. This leads to the so-called **likelihood equation**, also called

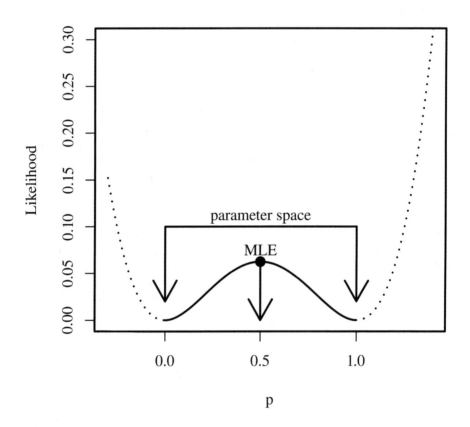

FIGURE 4.1
MLE as the maximum of the likelihood function over the parameter space. Dotted
parts of the function are outside the parameter space

the **score equation**,

$$\frac{d}{d\theta}\ell(\theta) = 0.$$

In most situations the MLE can be determined by solving this likelihood equation for θ. Often the log-likelihood function is a concave function, meaning that its second derivative is less than zero for all values of the parameter θ. In this case, if a solution to the likelihood equation can be found then it will be the unique MLE. We return to the importance of the second derivative of the log-likelihood function later on, where we will study its use in finding standard errors for MLEs.

In some cases the MLE cannot be calculated by solving the likelihood equation because the maximum of the log-likelihood function may not occur at a stationary point. This is often accompanied by the MLE being on the boundary of the parameter space, as illustrated in Example 4.2. These scenarios are less common but it is important to be aware of the possibility, and it may make it necessary to visually inspect the log-likelihood function. Further complexities associated with a non-stationary MLE will be discussed at the end of Section 4.4.

Example 4.2 The likelihood function for the fertility study discussed in Example 4.1 leads to the log-likelihood function

$$\ell(p) = n\log(p) + (y - n)\log(1 - p)$$

which has derivative

$$\frac{d}{dp}\ell(p) = \frac{n}{p} - \frac{y - n}{1 - p}.$$

Setting this derivative equal to zero and solving the resulting likelihood equation leads to the solution

$$\hat{p} = \frac{n}{y}$$

which is the MLE of p. Thus, for example, if there are $n = 2$ couples and $y = 4$ pregnancy attempts, then the MLE is $\hat{p} = 0.5$, as in Example 4.1. Recall that this approach to determining the MLE is only appropriate when the maximum of the log-likelihood is a stationary point. There is one situation in this type of study where the maximum of the log-likelihood does not occur at a stationary point, namely when all couples in the sample achieve pregnancy on their first cycle. In this case $y = n$ and the log-likelihood reduces to

$$\ell(p) = n\log(p)$$

which is plotted in Figure 4.2 for the case that $n = 2$. It is seen that there is no stationary point so the likelihood equation cannot be used to determine the MLE. From Figure 4.2, however, it can be seen clearly that the maximum of the log-likelihood function occurs at $\hat{p} = 1$, which is the MLE in this case. Coincidently this happens to be the same as the estimate that would have been obtained if we had applied the MLE that was derived based on the likelihood equation (since $y/n = 1$ when $y = n$). However, the justification for the MLE in this particular case has to come from Figure 4.2, rather than the likelihood equation. Note that the MLE corresponds to an estimate that all pregnancy attempts are successful. Although this is consistent with our particular sample, some statisticians would argue that this should be combined with our prior belief that there must at least be some chance of not getting pregnant, even if our particular sample does not reflect this. This is a called the Bayesian approach, to be discussed in Chapter 7, and would lead to an estimate that is less than 1.

In the previous example it was possible to solve the likelihood equation to get an expression for the MLE that can be evaluated given an observed sample. When this is possible we say that the MLE is **explicit**. In more complicated situations we may be able to write down the likelihood equation, but it may not be possible to solve it algebraically. When this occurs it is still possible to use maximum likelihood estimation, however, it will be necessary to use a computer to implement iterative algorithms to solve the likelihood equation numerically. We will not discuss such methods here, but note that practically all statistical software packages implement computational methods for numerically solving complicated likelihood equations. The most common examples of these techniques are the so-called **Fisher Scoring** and **Newton-Raphson** algorithms.

In very complicated situations, it may not even be possible to write down the derivative of the log-likelihood, in which case we would not be able to write down the likelihood equation. However, as long as we are able to evaluate the log-likelihood, it will usually be possible to implement an iterative algorithm on a computer, in order to numerically maximise the log-likelihood function. In such situations where we need to use a computer to numerically maximise the log-likelihood function, or equivalently solve the likelihood equation, we say that the MLE is **implicit**. Implicit MLEs are usually more difficult to calculate than explicit MLEs, and they may be more difficult to get an intuitive feel for since we do not have an algebraic expression that we can attempt to understand. Nonetheless, often the likelihood equation itself is of a form that can be used to gain an intuitive understanding of the MLE, as will be illustrated in the extended example. Furthermore, from a conceptual point of view, there is really no difference between explicit and implicit MLEs, in the sense that they both represent the parameter value that is most supported by the data through having the highest likelihood, regardless of the manner in which this value is calculated.

4.3   Information and standard errors

In order to calculate a standard error for the MLE, and hence to construct a confidence interval for the parameter based on the MLE, it is necessary to consider the variability of the MLE. From an intuitive point of view, we are likely to feel more confident about the parameter estimate based on the MLE if there is only a very narrow range of parameter values that achieve a likelihood value close to that achieved by the MLE. On the other hand, if there is a wide range of parameter values that achieve almost as

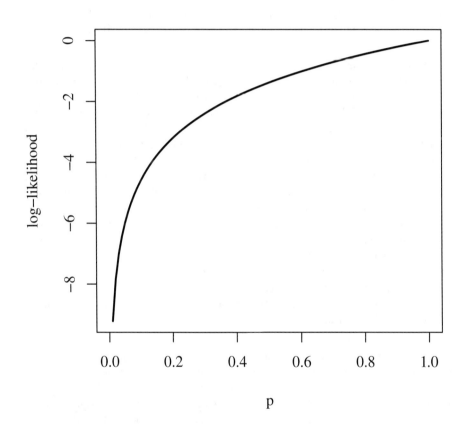

FIGURE 4.2
Log-likelihood function for the case where all pregnancy attempts were successful

high a likelihood as the MLE does, then we would not feel so confident in using the MLE to estimate the unknown parameter. In the latter situation, where a wide range of parameter values achieve almost as high a likelihood as the MLE, the likelihood function must be quite flat in the vicinity of the MLE. In the former situation, where a very narrow range of parameter values achieve likelihood values close to that of the MLE, the likelihood function must rise to a pronounced point in the vicinity of the MLE. This leads us to consider the curvature of the likelihood function, or equivalently the log-likelihood function, in the vicinity of the MLE, as an indication of the confidence that can be placed in the MLE for estimating the parameter. First we shall look at an illustration of this, and then subsequently we shall see how this curvature relates to the variance, and hence standard error, of the MLE.

Example 4.3 To see an example of the curvature of the likelihood function being greater when we are more confident about the MLE, consider two fertility samples that lead to the same MLE, namely $(n,y) = (2,4)$ and $(n,y) = (80,160)$. In both cases the MLE is $\hat{p} = 0.5$, however, with the substantially larger sample size in the second study we would have greater confidence in the MLE if we had observed the second sample than if we had observed the first sample. Figure 4.3 plots the two likelihood functions, based on the expression given in Example 4.1. Note that the scale of the vertical axis is the ratio of the likelihood function at each value of p, to the value at its maximum point. This allows the two plots to be compared on the same scale. It can be seen that for the first sample with $n = 2$ there is a much wider range of parameter values that achieve likelihood values close to that of the MLE, which is reflected in a flatter likelihood function. For the second sample with $n = 80$, where the curvature is much greater, the range of parameter values that achieve likelihood values close to that of the MLE is very narrow. This reflects much greater support for the MLE of $\hat{p} = 0.5$ based on the larger sample. We have expressed these plots in terms of the likelihood function, however, similar behaviour would have been observed on the log-likelihood scale also.

We have already seen how calculus can be useful for determining an MLE that occurs at a stationary point of a log-likelihood function. We now continue this discussion in the context of determining standard errors for MLEs. Calculus allows us to study the way in which functions vary. For example, the derivative of a function evaluated at a particular point tells us the rate of change, or gradient, of the function at that point. Likewise, the second derivative of a function, the derivative of the derivative, tells us the rate at which the gradient is changing. In the vicinity of the MLE, where a log-likelihood function achieves its maximum, its gradient will become progressively smaller, moving from being positive at parameter values that are less than the MLE, to being zero at the MLE, to being negative at parameter values greater than the MLE. This is indicative of the second derivative being negative. If the gradient is becoming progressively smaller at a very slow rate, then the log-likelihood function will be quite flat, and the second derivative will only be marginally less than zero. On the other hand, if the gradient is becoming progressively smaller at a fast

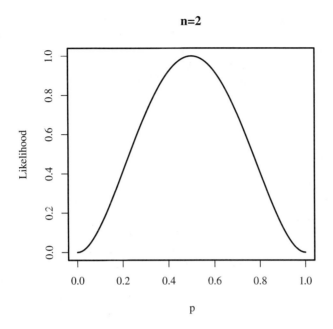

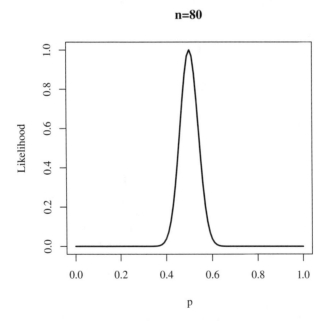

FIGURE 4.3
Two likelihood functions with the same MLE $\hat{p} = 0.5$ and different sample sizes

rate, then the log-likelihood function will be quite pointed, and the second derivative will be substantially less than zero. The extent to which the second derivative of
the log-likelihood function is less than zero is therefore a measure of the curvature
of the log-likelihood function. It seems natural therefore, that the magnitude of the
second derivative of the log-likelihood function at its maximum could be used as a
measure of the level of confidence that we can place in the MLE as an estimate of
the unknown parameter.

Consider the negative of the second derivative of the log-likelihood function,

$$I_O(\theta) = -\frac{d^2}{d\theta^2}\ell(\theta).$$

The quantity $I_O(\theta)$ depends on the observed sample through the dependence of the
log-likelihood function on the sample. We call $I_O(\theta)$ the **observed information** at
the parameter value θ. When evaluated at the MLE, $\theta = \hat{\theta}$, the observed information quantifies the curvature of the log-likelihood function at its maximum, and will
always be positive since, as discussed above, the second derivative is negative at the
MLE. Bearing in mind Figure 4.3, we can see that when $I_O(\hat{\theta})$ is "large" we will
have high confidence in the MLE as an estimate of the parameter, and when $I_O(\hat{\theta})$
is closer to zero we will have less confidence. This explains the use of the term "information", since $I_O(\hat{\theta})$ will be large when the data are very informative about the
parameter, and will be small when the data are less informative.

It turns out, however, that the observed information is much more than an intuitively sensible measure of the informativeness of the sample. The expectation of
the observed information is referred to as the **expected information**, or sometimes
the **Fisher information** after the statistician R.A. Fisher who first studied it. The
expected information is defined as

$$I(\theta) = \mathrm{E}\big[I_O(\theta;Y)\big]$$

and plays a crucial role in assessing the sampling variation of the MLE through the
relationship

$$\mathrm{Var}(\hat{\Theta}) \approx I(\theta)^{-1} \qquad \text{when } n \text{ is large.}$$

This approximation follows from a general asymptotic normality property of MLEs,
to be discussed in the next section. What it means is that if the information is large
then the variance of the MLE will be small, and if the information is small then the
variance of the MLE will be large. Based on the above asymptotic variance for the
MLE, a standard error based on the MLE in large samples can be calculated using
the quantity

$$\mathrm{SE}(\hat{\Theta}) = \sqrt{I(\hat{\theta})^{-1}}.$$

We will defer an example of the calculation of this standard error until the next
section where we discuss the calculation of confidence intervals based on the MLE.

4.4 Properties of the MLE

Until now we have relied on motivating the MLE by the intuition of choosing the parameter value that has greatest support from the data. In this section we use the desirable properties of estimators discussed in Chapter 2 to assess the usefulness of the MLE as an estimator. This section will focus on properties of the MLE that hold in the vast majority of cases, but at the end of the section we will consider some important, albeit uncommon, exceptions.

In general the MLE is not an unbiased estimator, although in specific circumstances the MLE may be unbiased. As an example it can be shown that for a normal distribution, such as the cholesterol modelling example we discussed in Chapters 2 and 3, the sample mean is the MLE of the population mean and so the MLE is unbiased. However, it turns out that for the same problem the sample variance dividing by n, S_n^2, is the MLE of σ^2 and so in this case the MLE is biased, as seen in the Chapter 2 exercises. While the MLE is not in general unbiased, it is a consistent estimator. Thus, asymptotically as $n \to \infty$ the MLE will end up coinciding with the true value of the parameter, and therefore satisfies the minimal desirable property that we would expect of any useful estimator. Furthermore, the asymptotic distribution of the MLE is a normal distribution, which is an additional desirable property that allows straightforward calculation of confidence intervals. In particular, using the variance that we discussed in the previous section, we have the following convergence in distribution property for an MLE

$$\sqrt{I(\theta)}\left(\hat{\Theta} - \theta\right) \xrightarrow{d} N(0,1).$$

This means that in large samples the sampling distribution of the MLE is approximately normal

$$\hat{\Theta} \stackrel{d}{\approx} N\left(\theta, I(\theta)^{-1}\right) \qquad \text{when } n \text{ is large.}$$

As discussed in Chapter 2, when the asymptotic variance of an estimator depends on the parameter we are trying to estimate, then we usually approximate the variance by substituting in the parameter estimate. This leads to the standard error of the MLE that we discussed in the previous section, and leads to a more useful approximate distribution for the MLE in large samples

$$\hat{\Theta} \stackrel{d}{\approx} N\left(\theta, I(\hat{\theta})^{-1}\right) \qquad \text{when } n \text{ is large.}$$

As a consequence of this asymptotic normality, confidence intervals for the parameter based on the MLE can be calculated using

$$\hat{\theta} \pm z_{1-\alpha/2}\sqrt{I(\hat{\theta})^{-1}}$$

where z_x is the x-percentile of the standard normal distribution (e.g. 1.96 for a 95% confidence interval).

Example 4.4 In this example we will use the fertility study setting to illustrate the calculation of a standard error for an MLE based on the expected information. In Example 4.2 we wrote down the derivative of the log-likelihood function for a sample involving observation of n couples having a total of y cycles to achieve pregnancy. Using the expression for $d\ell(p)/dp$ in Example 4.2, we can differentiate this again with respect to p to obtain the second derivative and hence the observed information

$$I_O(p;y) = -\frac{d^2}{dp^2}\ell(p) = -\left\{-\frac{n}{p^2} - \frac{y-n}{(1-p)^2}\right\}.$$

This leads to the expected information

$$I(p) = \mathrm{E}\left[I_O(p;Y)\right] = \frac{n}{p^2} + \frac{\mathrm{E}(Y) - n}{(1-p)^2}.$$

Using the fact that for a geometric distribution $\mathrm{E}(Y) = 1/p$, some algebra leads to

$$I(p) = \frac{n}{p^2(1-p)}.$$

A 95% confidence interval for the parameter p based on the MLE would therefore be

$$\frac{n}{y} \pm 1.96\sqrt{\frac{\hat{p}^2(1-\hat{p})}{n}}$$

which for the two scenarios in Example 4.3 would result in confidence intervals of $(0.01, 0.99)$ when the sample size is $n = 2$, and $(0.42, 0.58)$ when the sample size is $n = 80$. Notice that the width of these confidence intervals reflect a greater level of confidence in the MLE obtained from the larger study, as discussed in Example 4.3.

While the above desirable properties allow us to make use of the MLE and to have confidence that it is a sensible approach to estimation, they say nothing about how the MLE might compare with other approaches to estimation. In Chapter 2 we discussed the fact that there is a minimum possible asymptotic variance that a consistent estimator can have. Recalling this result from Chapter 2, and the fact that the log of the probability (density) function of the sample is identical to the log-likelihood function $\ell(\theta)$, it can be seen that the minimum possible asymptotic variance is equal to $I(\theta)^{-1}$. That is, the MLE has the smallest possible asymptotic variance of any consistent estimator. In the terminology introduced in Chapter 2, the MLE therefore has an asymptotic efficiency of 1, or is simply asymptotically efficient. This is a very important property, which means the MLE can be considered the **optimal estimator**. This is the primary motivation for recommending maximum likelihood as the best method of estimation for parametric models. Nonetheless, for a variety of reasons, such as insensitivity to outliers, it sometimes makes sense to consider other approaches to estimation. Some specific examples of such approaches have been studied in previous chapters and will be discussed further later in this chapter.

Finally, it is worth noting that although the desirable properties discussed above are true in the vast majority of situations, they do not hold in every situation where an MLE could be used as the parameter estimate. An important exception is when the MLE occurs on the boundary of the parameter space, such as in Example 4.2 when the MLE of the fertility proportion was estimated to be 1, which is the largest possible value that the parameter could take. In this case the asymptotic properties do not hold, and special techniques would be required to construct confidence intervals, depending on the particular situation. Another important exception arises in multiple parameter situations and will be discussed later in this chapter.

4.5 Parameter transformations

Sometimes we may be more interested in some function of a parameter, rather than the original parameter itself. For example, in epidemiology we sometimes study the prevalence odds of disease $\theta/(1-\theta)$, rather than the prevalence θ. The MLE has a further desirable property for estimating the function of a parameter. It turns out that for a transformation of the parameter, $g(\theta)$, the MLE of the transformed parameter is $g(\hat{\theta})$. Thus, for example, the MLE of the prevalence odds is $\hat{\theta}/(1-\hat{\theta})$. This property is called **invariance**, and means that we do not need to carry out a separate maximisation of the likelihood function if we change the scale on which the parameter is measured.

Although computation of the MLE of a transformed parameter $g(\theta)$ is straightforward if we already have the MLE of θ, computation of an associated standard error may not be so easy. Fortunately, there is a general method for computing approximate standard errors associated with $g(\hat{\theta})$, assuming that we already have a standard error associated with $\hat{\theta}$. This method is referred to as the **delta-method**.

One way to think about the delta-method is to consider the following approximation under the assumption that the transformation g has a derivative g'

$$g(\hat{\Theta}) \approx g(\theta) + g'(\theta)(\hat{\Theta} - \theta).$$

This is called a first order approximation of $g(\hat{\Theta})$, because it is the first part of the Taylor series expansion of $g(\hat{\Theta})$ about θ, and it will be accurate when $\hat{\Theta}$ is close to θ. Thus, given that $\hat{\Theta}$ is a consistent estimator of θ, this approximation will be accurate in large samples. Using this approximation, the delta-method for computing an approximate standard error comes from taking variances on both sides of the approximation, yielding

$$\mathrm{Var}\big[g(\hat{\Theta})\big] \approx g'(\theta)^2 \mathrm{Var}(\hat{\Theta})$$

giving the approximate standard error

$$\mathrm{se}\big[g(\hat{\theta})\big] \approx g'(\hat{\theta})\mathrm{se}(\hat{\theta}).$$

Notice that the approximate standard error associated with $g(\hat{\theta})$ depends on the standard error associated with $\hat{\theta}$ and the derivative of the parameter transformation. Thus, assuming we can can differentiate the transformation g, we can apply the delta-method whenever we have a standard error associated with $\hat{\theta}$.

As well as an approximate standard error, the delta-method also yields an approximate normal distribution for the transformed estimator. The justification for this comes from a result in probability theory saying that if $\hat{\Theta}$ is asymptotically normally distributed then $g(\hat{\Theta})$ is asymptotically normally distributed, again assuming that g can be differentiated. This leads to the approximate normal distribution

$$g(\hat{\Theta}) \overset{d}{\approx} N\left(g(\theta), \mathrm{se}\left[g(\hat{\theta})\right]^2 \right) \qquad \text{when } n \text{ is large.}$$

This approximate normality can be used to construct confidence intervals for the transformed parameter in large samples, as illustrated in the following example.

Example 4.5 Consider a disease prevalence study where the observed number of individuals with the disease of interest y, from a random sample of n individuals, is modelled as the observed value of a random variable Y with binomial distribution $Y \overset{d}{=} \mathrm{Bin}(n, \theta)$. As discussed in Example 2.5 of Chapter 2, a standard error associated with the estimate $\hat{\theta} = y/n$ is

$$\mathrm{se}(\hat{\theta}) = \sqrt{\frac{\hat{\theta}(1-\hat{\theta})}{n}}$$

which leads to the 95% confidence interval for the disease prevalence, $\hat{\theta} \pm 1.96\mathrm{se}(\hat{\theta})$. Notice that this confidence interval can potentially include values that are outside the range $[0,1]$, which does not make sense given that θ is a probability. This disadvantage can be rectified by choosing an appropriate transformation of the parameter θ. A common transformation of probabilities, such as the disease prevalence θ, is the log-odds transformation

$$g(\theta) = \log\left(\frac{\theta}{1-\theta} \right).$$

Notice that this transformed parameter is unrestricted, since it can range from $-\infty$ to $+\infty$ as θ ranges from 0 to 1. Given the standard error $\mathrm{se}(\hat{\theta})$ for the prevalence, the delta-method can be used to construct an approximate standard error and confidence interval for the prevalence log-odds. First, we need to differentiate the transformation

$$g'(\theta) = \frac{1}{\theta(1-\theta)}.$$

This then leads to the approximate standard error

$$\mathrm{se}\left[g(\hat{\theta})\right] \approx \frac{1}{\hat{\theta}(1-\hat{\theta})} \sqrt{\frac{\hat{\theta}(1-\hat{\theta})}{n}} = \sqrt{\frac{1}{n\hat{\theta}(1-\hat{\theta})}}$$

and the 95% confidence interval for the prevalence log-odds, $g(\hat{\theta}) \pm 1.96\mathrm{se}\left[g(\hat{\theta})\right]$.

One of the reasons for using the delta-method is that the approximate normality required to construct a confidence interval may be more accurate on a transformed parameter scale. This is particularly true for situations like that discussed in Example 4.5, where the parameter is restricted to a particular range but where the transformed parameter is not restricted to any particular range. In such cases the normal approximation is often better for the transformed parameter because normally distributed random variables are not restricted to any particular range. We return to this issue in Section 4.8.6 and the exercises.

It should be noted that the delta-method is not limited to MLEs. If the estimate $\hat{\theta}$ has been derived using some other method of estimation, such as those discussed in Section 4.7, the standard error associated with $g(\hat{\theta})$ can still be obtained using the delta-method. However, together with the invariance property of MLEs, the delta-method is particularly useful for MLEs, because it leads to an approximate standard error associated with the MLE of the transformed parameter $g(\theta)$.

4.6 Multiple parameters

When our parametric model involves more than one parameter, $\theta = (\theta_1, \ldots, \theta_p)$, maximum likelihood estimation may become more complicated, however, similar properties to those discussed above will continue to hold. The first point to note when we have more than one parameter is that instead of a single likelihood equation, we now have a collection of p **likelihood equations** or **score equations**. These equations are obtained by partial differentiation of the log-likelihood with respect to each parameter, which is carried out by differentiating with respect to each parameter separately, while treating the other parameters as constants. According to standard calculus notation, partial differentiation is denoted using the symbol ∂ in place of d in univariable differentiation, leading to the likelihood equations

$$\frac{\partial}{\partial \theta_1} \ell(\theta_1, \ldots, \theta_p) = 0$$

$$\vdots$$

$$\frac{\partial}{\partial \theta_p} \ell(\theta_1, \ldots, \theta_p) = 0.$$

These are a collection of p simultaneous equations that need to be solved to give the p parameter estimates $\hat{\theta} = (\hat{\theta}_1, \ldots, \hat{\theta}_p)$. According to standard multivariable calculus, this will lead to maximisation of the multivariable log-likelihood function.

As in the one parameter case, when there are multiple parameters the MLE is consistent and asymptotically normal. This normal distribution will be a multivariate normal distribution, with a variance-covariance matrix that depends on an information matrix. In particular, let

$$I_{ij} = \frac{\partial^2}{\partial \theta_i \partial \theta_j} \ell(\theta_1, \ldots, \theta_p),$$

that is, the derivative of the log-likelihood function first with respect to θ_j (treating the other parameters as constants) and then again with respect to θ_i (treating the other parameters as constants). We can then define the **observed information matrix** as the $p \times p$ matrix $I_O(\theta) = [I_{ij}]$. This leads to the **expected information matrix** $I(\theta) = \mathrm{E}[I_O(\theta)]$, which is obtained by taking the expectation of each element of the observed information matrix. The asymptotic distribution of the MLE can then be written down analogously to the one parameter case. This leads to the approximate distribution

$$\hat{\Theta} \overset{d}{\approx} \mathrm{N}_p(\theta, I(\hat{\theta})^{-1}) \qquad \text{when } n \text{ is large.}$$

The large sample distribution of the MLE of multiple parameters is a generalisation of the large sample distribution discussed in the one parameter case. Notice in particular that since θ is a p-dimensional vector, the large sample distribution of the MLE has a p-dimensional multivariate normal distribution, which was discussed in Chapter 1 and is also summarised in Appendix 1. Furthermore, the inverse of the expected information, $I(\theta)^{-1}$, is now a matrix inverse rather than a reciprocal. This leads to a (symmetric) $p \times p$ matrix that becomes the variance-covariance matrix in the multivariate normal distribution. Standard errors associated with each $\hat{\theta}_i$ are obtained from the corresponding diagonal elements of the inverse of the information matrix, after substituting in the parameter estimate $\hat{\theta}$. Thus, the standard error associated with $\hat{\theta}_i$ is the square root of the (i,i) element of $I(\hat{\theta})^{-1}$, which can be used to construct a confidence interval as in the one parameter case. The extended example includes a detailed illustration of this process.

There is an important exception to the consistency and asymptotic normality of MLEs in multiple parameter situations. This exception arises when the number of parameters increases as the sample size increases. Occasionally a model may be proposed in which p is equal to the sample size n, or at least increases as the sample size increases. In such cases the MLE is usually not consistent and asymptotically normal. Thus, in practice it may be questionable to rely on the MLE when the number of parameters is as large, or almost as large, as the number of observations in the sample. In such situations a simpler model may be required, or possibly a larger sample.

4.7   Further estimation methods

Maximum likelihood estimation is the most commonly used general method of estimation. It is applicable to any situation in which we have a likelihood function corresponding to a parametric model, and it is the most efficient method of estimation in large samples. Nonetheless, there are other approaches to estimation. While none of these methods is as generally applicable as maximum likelihood estimation, alternative approaches can be useful in specific contexts.

4.7.1   Least squares estimation

Perhaps the most important alternative to maximum likelihood estimation is the method of **least squares estimation**. Whereas maximum likelihood estimation chooses the estimate that maximises the likelihood associated with the observed sample, least squares estimation chooses the estimate that minimises the discrepancy between the sample observations and the estimated sample means.

As a simple introduction, consider a sample of observations $y_1, \ldots, y_n$, which are the observed values of random variables $Y_1, \ldots, Y_n$ with $E(Y_i) = \mu$, for all $i = 1, \ldots, n$. A measure of the discrepancy between observation i and the mean μ is $(y_i - \mu)^2$, since this will be large when y_i is far away from μ and close to zero when y_i is close to μ. Aggregating over all of the observations leads to an overall measure of the discrepancy between the sample and μ, namely, the **sum of squares**

$$SS(\mu) = \sum_{i=1}^{n} (y_i - \mu)^2.$$

The least squares estimate $\tilde{\mu}$ is then defined as the value of μ that minimises $SS(\mu)$, that is, the value of μ that minimises the overall discrepancy between the sample observations and the estimated mean.

Computation of the least squares estimate then involves minimisation of the function $SS(\mu)$ which can be achieved using calculus. In particular, this involves solving the least squares **estimating equation**

$$\frac{d}{d\mu} SS(\mu) = -2 \sum_{i=1}^{n} (y_i - \mu) = 0$$

which gives the least squares estimate $\tilde{\mu} = \bar{y}$. As for the MLE, the corresponding least squares estimator uses the same definition applied to the random variables $Y_1, \ldots, Y_n$. That is, the least squares estimator is $\tilde{M} = \bar{Y}$.

Notice that the derivation of the least squares estimator did not make use of the distribution of the sample. This is both an advantage and a disadvantage compared to maximum likelihood estimation. It is an advantage because it means that the least squares approach is applicable in the same form for all distributions, unlike maximum likelihood which uses a different likelihood function for different distributions. On the other hand, this can be a disadvantage because the form of the distribution can provide additional information that can provide greater estimation efficiency. This means that when maximum likelihood estimation and least squares estimation produce different estimators, the MLE will be more efficient than the least squares estimator. Sometimes though, the two approaches will produce the same estimator. In particular, when the sample has a normal distribution, then the two approaches will coincide because the log-likelihood for a normal distribution is simply the negative of the sum of squares.

The simple illustrative presentation above can be generalised to a parameter vector $\theta = (\theta_1, \ldots, \theta_p)$, with $E(Y_i) = \mu_i(\theta)$. In this case the sum of squares is

$$SS(\theta_1, \ldots, \theta_p) = \sum_{i=1}^{n} \left[y_i - \mu_i(\theta) \right]^2$$

which leads to the p least squares estimating equations

$$\frac{\partial}{\partial \theta_1} SS(\theta_1, \ldots, \theta_p) = 0$$

$$\vdots$$

$$\frac{\partial}{\partial \theta_p} SS(\theta_1, \ldots, \theta_p) = 0.$$

These p simultaneous equations must be solved for the least squares estimate $\tilde{\theta} = (\tilde{\theta}_1, \ldots, \tilde{\theta}_p)$, just like the likelihood equations are solved to find the MLE.

The most common application of least squares estimation is linear regression analysis. In linear regression analysis the sample $Y_1, \ldots, Y_n$ is assumed to have a normal distribution $Y_i \overset{d}{=} N(\mu_i, \sigma^2)$, where the means μ_i are taken to be linear functions of covariates that differ between observations. For example, if we were interested in assessing the relationship between cholesterol level Y_i and blood pressure x_i using a sample of $i = 1, \ldots, n$ individuals, μ_i would take the linear form

$$\mu_i(\theta) = \theta_1 + \theta_2 x_i \qquad i = 1, \ldots, n$$

and $\theta = (\theta_1, \theta_2)$ would be estimated by minimising the sum of squares $SS(\theta_1, \theta_2)$. The least squares estimate $\tilde{\theta}_2$ would then provide information about the extent to which cholesterol level increases as blood pressure increases. A detailed discussion of linear regression is beyond the scope of this book, but further reading on related topics is discussed in Appendix 3, including a chapter in the book by Kleinbaum et al. (2008) on the correspondence between least squares and maximum likelihood estimation for linear regression with a normal distribution model.

Another possible application of least squares estimation is where it is more convenient than maximum likelihood estimation, such as situations where the MLE is implicit but the least squares estimate is explicit. An example of this sort of situation is considered in the exercises.

4.7.2   Method of moments estimation

The discussion of least squares estimation in Section 4.7.1 introduced us to the idea that there are other general approaches to deriving estimation procedures beyond maximum likelihood estimation. In fact, there are many other general approaches, some of which we briefly note here.

For a parameter vector $\theta = (\theta_1, \ldots, \theta_p)$, recall that both maximum likelihood and least squares estimation are based on a collection of p simultaneous equations that must be solved to produce estimates of the p parameters. We use the general term **estimating equations** to refer to the collection of equations that must be solved to calculate the estimates. Another method of estimation, called the **method of moments**, uses a different approach to construct the p estimating equations that must be solved to provide the estimates. This approach is based on the concepts of a sample moment and a distribution moment, which are generalisations of the concepts of a sample mean and a distribution mean. In particular, consider the random variables $Y_1, \ldots, Y_n$, all with the same distribution, and let the observed values be $y_1, \ldots, y_n$. Then the kth sample moment and the kth distribution moment are respectively

$$m^{(k)} = \frac{1}{n}\sum_{i=1}^{n} y_i^k \quad \text{and} \quad \mu^{(k)}(\theta_1, \ldots, \theta_p) = \mathrm{E}\left(Y_i^k\right) \quad k = 1, 2, \ldots .$$

It can be seen that these two definitions of moments generalise the concept of a mean, in the sense that in both cases the mean is obtained by taking $k = 1$.

The method of moments chooses the estimate that ensures the sample moments are equal to the estimated distribution moments. This ensures that the estimated distribution matches the sample in some sense. Since p simultaneous equations are required when there are p parameters, method of moments estimation uses the first p moments, and involves solving the equations

$$\mu^{(1)}(\theta_1, \ldots, \theta_p) = m^{(1)}$$
$$\vdots$$
$$\mu^{(p)}(\theta_1, \ldots, \theta_p) = m^{(p)}.$$

Like least squares estimation, for some models the method of moments will produce the same estimate as maximum likelihood estimation, and for other models it will produce a different estimate. Often it turns out that method of moments estimates are explicit estimates in situations where the MLE is implicit, which often makes them more convenient to calculate. However, like least squares estimation, method of moments estimation tends to be inefficient relative to maximum likelihood estimation.

Example 4.6 A simple example of method of moments estimation is for a sample $y_1, \ldots, y_n$ from random variables $Y_1, \ldots, Y_n$ with $Y_i \overset{d}{=} \mathrm{N}(\mu, \sigma^2)$. Then $\mu^{(1)} = \mu$ and $\mu^{(2)} = \sigma^2 + \mu^2$ so that the method of moments estimates are the solution of the two estimating equations

$$\mu = \bar{y}$$
$$\sigma^2 + \mu^2 = \frac{1}{n}\sum_{i=1}^{n} y_i^2.$$

Solving these two equations gives the method of moments estimates $\tilde{\mu} = \bar{y}$ and $\tilde{\sigma}^2 = s_n^2$, which are identical to the MLEs. Some further examples of method of moments estimation are considered in the exercises.

4.7.3 Modified likelihoods

Finally, it is important to note that we have already seen the basis for alternatives to maximum likelihood estimation when we discussed modified versions of the likelihood function that deal with nuisance parameters, in Section 3.6. The main modified version of the likelihood that was discussed in Section 3.6 was the profile likelihood, which provides a method for eliminating nuisance parameters from the likelihood function, leaving only the parameters of interest. The profile likelihood, and other modified versions of the likelihood function mentioned in Section 3.6, can be used as the basis of estimation and confidence interval construction, in much the same way as the likelihood function is used with maximum likelihood estimation. Thus, once the profile likelihood has been determined, for example as illustrated in Section 3.7.5, then it can be maximised to produce parameter estimates and its second derivative matrix can be used to construct standard errors and confidence intervals. This can have the advantage of being more straightforward than maximum likelihood estimation, because the nuisance parameters are eliminated from the estimation process, while at the same time having the same efficiency as the MLE in large samples. We will discuss the profile likelihood further in the extended example, in Section 4.8.4, and also consider it further in the exercises.

4.8 Extended example

In Chapter 3 we discussed the development of likelihood functions for a Poisson model of stroke incidence among individuals with coronary disease, and its relationship with salt intake. In this extended example the objective is to continue the discussion to show how to use these likelihood functions to derive the MLE of the stroke incidence rate and rate ratio, and how to use the concept of information to obtain standard errors and confidence intervals. We start by discussing the one parameter situation, where it is assumed that there is no difference between high and low salt intake populations with regard to stroke incidence. The multiple parameter situation is then considered for maximum likelihood estimation of the rate ratio and individual exposure group rates, including a discussion of the likelihood equations and information matrix. We will then use this to draw conclusions about whether there is evidence that stroke rates differ between the two salt intake groups.

4.8.1 Modelling stroke incidence

We will rely on the same notation and model that was used in the Chapter 3 extended example. In particular, we will assume that our sample $Y = (Y_1, Y_2)$ corresponds to the number of new cases of stroke in the high salt intake and low salt intake exposure groups, respectively. For concreteness we will discuss a study in which the observed sample is $y = (y_1, y_2) = (245, 239)$, based on a sample size of $(n_1, n_2) = (1150, 850)$

individuals having been followed for a total of $(F_1, F_2) = (5980, 3825)$ person years. The stroke incidence rates in the two groups are denoted by (λ_1, λ_2), with rate ratio $\gamma = \lambda_2/\lambda_1$, and the distribution of Y_i is Poisson($\lambda_i F_i$).

4.8.2 MLE for a common stroke rate

In the one parameter context where a common stroke rate $\lambda = \lambda_1 = \lambda_2$ is assumed for the two salt exposure groups, then the likelihood function and log-likelihood function that were written down in Chapter 3 are (omitting irrelevant terms that do not depend on λ)

$$L(\lambda) = \lambda^{y_1+y_2} \exp\left[-(F_1+F_2)\lambda\right]$$

and

$$\ell(\lambda) = (y_1+y_2)\log\lambda - (F_1+F_2)\lambda.$$

Differentiation of $\ell(\lambda)$ yields the likelihood equation

$$\frac{d}{d\lambda}\ell(\lambda) = \frac{y_1+y_2}{\lambda} - (F_1+F_2) = 0.$$

Solving this likelihood equation leads to the MLE

$$\hat{\lambda} = \frac{y_1+y_2}{F_1+F_2}$$

which takes the value $\hat{\lambda} = 0.0494$. In Chapter 3 we noted that this parameter value was the most supported value of any parameter value. The above discussion illustrates why this is the case, namely, because it solves the likelihood equation and hence maximises the likelihood function. Note that the parameter λ represents the rate at which individuals experience a stroke, per year. Thus, λ must be non-negative for our model to make sense, and the parameter space consists of the values $\lambda \geq 0$. The MLE described above can never be negative, and will provide the parameter value with the highest value of the likelihood function among all non-negative values. It is, however, possible to evaluate the likelihood function $L(\lambda)$ at negative values of λ, even though they have no meaningful interpretation in terms of our stroke incidence model. This highlights the fact that maximisation of the likelihood function, or log-likelihood function, should be conducted within the parameter space only. For a Poisson distribution the likelihood function can take on greater values outside the parameter space, however, it does not have a likelihood interpretation for such parameter values and is of no relevance in determining the MLE. In general, if a solution to the likelihood equation falls inside the parameter space then it will be the MLE. For some models (not including the current one) it may be possible for a solution to the likelihood equation to fall outside the parameter space, in which case it cannot be used as the MLE. This is uncommon but when it occurs care needs to be taken and the log-likelihood function may need to be inspected graphically.

4.8.3   Confidence interval for a common stroke rate

To calculate a confidence interval for the stroke incidence rate, we first need to derive the expected information, based on the second derivative of the log-likelihood. The first derivative of the log-likelihood was used above in the likelihood equation, and this can be differentiated again with respect to λ, leading to the observed information

$$I_O(\lambda;y) = -\frac{d^2}{d\lambda^2}\ell(\lambda) = \frac{y_1 + y_2}{\lambda^2}.$$

Using the fact that $E(Y_i) = \lambda F_i$, the expected information is given by

$$I(\lambda) = E\left[I_O(\lambda;Y)\right] = \frac{\lambda F_1 + \lambda F_2}{\lambda^2} = \frac{F_1 + F_2}{\lambda}.$$

Using $\sqrt{I(\hat{\lambda})^{-1}}$ as a standard error for the MLE leads to the following 95% confidence interval for the stroke incidence rate,

$$\frac{y_1 + y_2}{F_1 + F_2} \pm 1.96\sqrt{\frac{\hat{\lambda}}{F_1 + F_2}}.$$

For the particular sample considered above this corresponds to a 95% confidence interval of $(0.045, 0.054)$ for the common stroke incidence rate, per person per year.

4.8.4   MLE for the rate ratio

If we remove the assumption of a common stroke incidence rate then the log-likelihood function becomes a function of two parameters, λ_1 and λ_2. In Chapter 3 we discussed how to use the reparameterisation $\lambda_2 = \gamma\lambda_1$ to write the log-likelihood function as a function of both the stroke incidence rate in the high salt group, λ_1, and the ratio of the stroke incidence rates in the two groups, γ. This leads to the log-likelihood function

$$\ell(\lambda_1, \gamma) = y_1 \log \lambda_1 + y_2 \log(\gamma\lambda_1) - F_1\lambda_1 - F_2\gamma\lambda_1.$$

This function can be differentiated with respect to λ_1 (treating γ as a constant) and with respect to γ (treating λ_1 as a constant). This leads to the following likelihood equations

$$\frac{\partial}{\partial\lambda_1}\ell(\lambda_1, \gamma) = \frac{y_1 + y_2}{\lambda_1} - F_1 - F_2\gamma = 0$$

$$\frac{\partial}{\partial\gamma}\ell(\lambda_1, \gamma) = \frac{y_2}{\gamma} - F_2\lambda_1 = 0.$$

These are simultaneous equations that must be solved to obtain the MLE $(\hat{\lambda}_1, \hat{\gamma})$. By rearranging each of the two likelihood equations we obtain the following two simultaneous equations

$$\hat{\lambda}_1 = \frac{y_1 + y_2}{F_1 + \hat{\gamma}F_2}$$

$$\hat{\lambda}_1 = \frac{y_2}{\hat{\gamma}F_2}$$

and setting these two equations equal to each other and solving for $\hat{\gamma}$ leads to

$$\hat{\gamma} = \frac{y_2/F_2}{y_1/F_1} = 1.52.$$

Although we are most interested in the rate ratio in the present example, as a by-product we also obtain

$$\hat{\lambda}_1 = \frac{y_1}{F_1} = 0.0410.$$

These estimates are of course the natural estimates, and justify our use of these estimates in Chapter 3. In particular, in Chapter 3 we found that $\hat{\gamma} = 1.52$ is the most supported value of all values for the rate ratio, based on the profile log-likelihood, a result that is consistent with it being the MLE. Recall also that in our discussion of the profile log-likelihood for γ, we had to take as given that the most supported value of λ_1 for any given value of γ is equal to

$$\hat{\lambda}_1(\gamma) = \frac{y_1 + y_2}{F_1 + \gamma F_2}.$$

Notice that this result comes from solving the likelihood equations, and corresponds to the first of the two simplified simultaneous equations above.

In this section we have derived the rate ratio estimate by maximising the full likelihood function, which involves simultaneously estimating λ_1. If we are only interested in the rate ratio and not λ_1, another approach would be to maximise the profile likelihood discussed in Chapter 3. This involves first eliminating the nuisance parameter λ_1, and then maximising the profile likelihood as a function of γ alone. In the exercises we will see that for this model this leads to identical estimates of γ. In general, if we are truly not interested in estimating the nuisance parameter then a profile likelihood approach may be preferable because it avoids unnecessary estimation of the nuisance parameter. However, for this example we will continue with standard error estimation for both parameters, as an illustration of a multi-dimensional context, and defer consideration of the profile likelihood approach until the exercises.

4.8.5 Confidence interval for the rate ratio

To obtain a confidence interval for the rate ratio we first need to obtain the expected information matrix based on the two-parameter log-likelihood function. This requires us to differentiate the two derivatives that appear in the likelihood equations, each with respect to both parameters, thus yielding four second derivatives that make up a 2×2 matrix. Below we write down each of the four elements that make up the observed information matrix $I_O(\lambda_1, \gamma) = [I_{ij}]$:

$$I_{11} = -\frac{\partial^2}{\partial \lambda_1^2} \ell(\lambda_1, \gamma) = \frac{y_1 + y_2}{\lambda_1^2}$$

$$I_{21} = I_{12} = -\frac{\partial^2}{\partial \gamma \partial \lambda_1} \ell(\lambda_1, \gamma) = -\frac{\partial^2}{\partial \lambda_1 \partial \gamma} \ell(\lambda_1, \gamma) = F_2$$

$$I_{22} = -\frac{\partial^2}{\partial \gamma^2} \ell(\lambda_1, \gamma) = \frac{y_2}{\gamma^2}.$$

By using the fact that $E(Y_i) = \lambda F_i$, and taking the expectation of each element of the observed information matrix listed above, we obtain the expected information matrix

$$I(\lambda_1, \gamma) = \begin{bmatrix} \frac{F_1 + \gamma F_2}{\lambda_1} & F_2 \\ F_2 & \frac{\lambda_1 F_2}{\gamma} \end{bmatrix}.$$

For our particular sample, substituting in the values of $\hat{\gamma}$ and $\hat{\lambda}_1$ allows us to evaluate this expected information matrix

$$I(\hat{\lambda}_1, \hat{\gamma}) = \begin{bmatrix} 287658.5 & 3825 \\ 3825 & 103.17 \end{bmatrix}$$

and its matrix inverse

$$I(\hat{\lambda}_1, \hat{\gamma})^{-1} = \begin{bmatrix} 6.86 \times 10^{-6} & -2.54 \times 10^{-4} \\ -2.54 \times 10^{-4} & 0.0191 \end{bmatrix}.$$

Our primary interest lies in the rate ratio MLE $\hat{\gamma}$, for which a standard error is obtained by taking the corresponding diagonal element of the inverse of the expected information matrix, namely $\sqrt{0.0191} = 0.138$. This leads to a 95% confidence interval

$$1.52 \pm 1.96 \times 0.138 = (1.25, 1.79).$$

In the Chapter 3 extended example we noted that unequal stroke rates were more supported by the data than equal rates, with the most supported value for the stroke rate ratio being 1.52. At that stage, however, we were not in a position to assess whether there was "significant" evidence against the proposition that the stroke rates in the two groups are equal. Based on the above confidence interval we are now in a position to assess this. In particular, it can be seen that based on the confidence interval, a rate ratio value of 1 is not plausible since it does not lie inside the confidence interval. This indicates that there is evidence of a significantly higher stroke rate in the group exposed to a high salt diet, and introduces us to the idea of hypothesis testing, which will be studied in some detail in the coming chapters.

4.8.6 Reparameterisation

Although the confidence intervals derived above are valid when the sample size is large, it sometimes makes sense to calculate confidence intervals after expressing the parameters on a transformed scale. An example of this in the present context would be to transform the parameters, or reparameterise, so that the model is expressed in terms of the log incidence rates and the log incidence rate ratio. For the single parameter situation discussed at the beginning of the chapter, if we were to reparameterise by writing $\theta = \log \lambda$ then the log-likelihood function could be rewritten in terms of θ instead of λ. Maximisation of this reparameterised log-likelihood would lead to the MLE $\hat{\theta} = \log \hat{\lambda}$, where $\hat{\lambda}$ was defined earlier in this extended example. This is consistent with the property of invariance of the MLE that we noted earlier in this chapter, and means that estimation is effectively equivalent whether carried out on the transformed or original scale. However, a confidence interval for θ based on the expected information from the reparameterised log-likelihood would not lead to the same confidence interval for λ as that used previously in this extended example. In particular, if the confidence interval for θ obtained using the expected information from the reparameterised log-likelihood is $(\hat{\theta}_L, \hat{\theta}_U)$, then a corresponding confidence interval for λ can be obtained using $(\exp \hat{\theta}_L, \exp \hat{\theta}_U)$. The question then arises: why would we want to carry out our confidence interval calculation based on a transformed parameter rather than on the original scale? One of the reasons for doing this is that the normal approximation may be more applicable in smaller sample sizes when the parameters are appropriately transformed, than when they are left on their original scale. Thus, the confidence interval for λ may be more accurate when based on the transformed parameter. We will consider this issue further in the exercises. For certain types of distributions there are particular transformations or reparameterisations that work best. For example, in the case of the Poisson distribution it is the log transformation of the parameter that works best. This issue is related to the topic of generalised linear models, which are generalisations of linear regression that lead to linear models for a transformation of the mean, rather than the mean itself. Such models are beyond our scope, but further reading can be found in such books as Dobson and Barnett (2008) and other texts discussed in Appendix 3. Although confidence intervals for appropriately transformed parameters may be more accurate in smaller sample sizes, when the sample is sufficiently large then confidence intervals will be similar, whether based on transformed or untransformed parameters.

Exercises

1. In Chapter 3 we considered a series of examples in which we discussed likelihood functions for a disease prevalence study, based on the binomial distribution.

   (a) Review these examples and write down the likelihood function and log-likelihood function for the population prevalence θ, in terms of the number of individuals in the sample n, and the number of individuals in the sample who have the disease y.

   (b) Using differentiation, write down the likelihood equation.

(c) Based on the likelihood equation determine $\hat{\theta}$, the MLE of θ. Hence justify that the sample prevalence is the best estimate of the population prevalence.

(d) Determine the expected information, in terms of θ and n.

(e) Using part (d), evaluate standard errors associated with the MLE, for the two samples discussed in Example 3.2 of Chapter 3. Hence calculate confidence intervals for the population prevalence based on each of these samples.

2. Read the section on reparameterisation in the extended example and review the log-likelihood function for the case of a common stroke rate λ. Let $\theta = \log \lambda$. We will now consider the likelihood and MLE based on this transformed parameter.

(a) Using the log-likelihood for λ write down the log-likelihood function as a function of θ, by substituting in $\theta = \log \lambda$.

(b) Using the log-likelihood in part (a), write down the likelihood equation for θ and hence determine $\hat{\theta}$ the MLE of θ.

(c) Verify that $\hat{\theta} = \log \hat{\lambda}$, where $\hat{\lambda}$ is the MLE that was derived in the extended example. This is an example of what general property of MLEs?

(d) After differentiating the left-hand side of the likelihood equation, obtain the expected information. For the sample described in the extended example, use the expected information to calculate a standard error based on $\hat{\theta}$, and hence a confidence interval for θ.

(e) Using part (d), calculate a confidence interval for λ and compare this confidence interval with the one that was calculated in the extended example.

(f) Consider the two approaches to calculating confidence intervals in part (e). Would it be possible (in other samples) for either of these two approaches to yield confidence intervals that include values outside the parameter space? Which approach is more desirable from this point of view?

3. In this question we return to the systolic blood pressure lowering study described in Exercise 6 of Chapter 2. Begin by reviewing that exercise. For the current exercise, we will assume that the population standard deviation reduction in systolic blood pressure is known to be 12 mmHg, so that $\sigma^2 = 144$. Of course, in practice it is unrealistic to assume that we know the standard deviation exactly, however, we will consider the case where the standard deviation is not known in Exercise 5.

(a) Write down the log-likelihood function for the single parameter, the population mean μ.

(b) Using differentiation write down the likelihood equation.

(c) Based on the likelihood equation determine $\hat{\mu}$, the MLE of μ.

(d) Determine the expected information, and hence write down a 95% confidence interval for μ, in terms of the sample mean $\bar{y}$.

4. This question deals with multiple parameter MLEs for the fertility study example, and follows the same type of approach as was used in the extended example for stroke incidence rates. Review Exercise 8 from Chapter 3, for the fertility study where women who are smokers have different fertility to women who are non-smokers. In that exercise we studied a likelihood function that was a function of two parameters, the fertility parameter for women who smoke (p_2), and the relative fertility rate (γ). Start by writing down the log-likelihood function from part (b) of that exercise.

(a) Differentiate the log-likelihood with respect to p_2 to obtain the first likelihood equation. Then differentiate the log-likelihood with respect to γ to obtain the second likelihood equation.

(b) Rearrange both likelihood equations so that p_2 is on the left-hand side. Hence solve the likelihood equations to obtain the MLEs of p_2 and γ. Based on these MLEs, what will the MLE of p_1 be?

(c) Differentiate the left-hand side of each likelihood equation with respect to p_2. Then differentiate the left-hand side of each likelihood equation with respect to γ. Hence write down the observed information matrix, and take the expectation of this to obtain the expected information matrix.

(d) For the data set described in Exercise 7 of Chapter 3, evaluate each of the elements in the expected information matrix, by substituting in the MLEs of the parameters. Take the matrix inverse of the expected information matrix, and hence obtain a standard error and a confidence interval for γ.

(e) Based on part (d), is there evidence that fertility differs between women who smoke and women who are non-smokers?

5. This question is a continuation of Exercise 3, but now we make the more realistic assumption that the population variance of the reduction in systolic blood pressure is not known.

(a) Write down the log-likelihood function for the parameters μ and σ^2.

(b) Write down the two likelihood equations.

(c) Solve the likelihood equations to determine the MLEs of μ and σ^2.

(d) Based on your answer in part (c), what would be the MLE of σ (give reasons)?

(e) Determine the expected information matrix, and also its matrix inverse, in terms of μ and σ^2.

(f) Based on your answer in part (e), write down a 95% confidence interval for μ.

(g) How does the confidence interval in part (f) differ from the first confidence interval described in Exercise 6 of Chapter 2? Which confidence interval would have higher coverage probability?

6. Consider the disease prevalence study discussed in Exercise 1, where the observed number of individuals with the disease of interest y, from a random sample of n individuals, is modelled as the observed value of a random variable Y with binomial distribution $Y \stackrel{d}{=} \text{Bin}(n, \theta)$. In this question we will consider the population prevalence θ, as well as the prevalence log-odds ϕ, the log prevalence β and the prevalence odds γ, where

$$\phi = \log\left(\frac{\theta}{1-\theta}\right) \qquad \beta = \log(\theta) \qquad \gamma = \frac{\theta}{1-\theta}.$$

(a) Write down the MLE of the population prevalence $\hat{\theta}$ and a standard error $\text{se}(\hat{\theta})$.

(b) By referring back to Example 4.5, write down the MLE of the prevalence log-odds $\hat{\phi}$ and a standard error $\text{se}(\hat{\phi})$ obtained using the delta-method.

(c) Using the same approach as Example 4.5, write down the MLEs of the log prevalence $\hat{\beta}$ and the prevalence odds $\hat{\gamma}$, as well as standard errors $\text{se}(\hat{\beta})$ and $\text{se}(\hat{\gamma})$, obtained using the delta-method.

(d) Consider samples where $n = 20$ and $n = 100$. In each case suppose that 10% of individuals in the sample have the disease of interest. Compute confidence intervals for each of the 4 parameters θ, ϕ, β and γ, for each of the 2 sample sizes.

(e) Repeat part (d) supposing that 90% of individuals in the sample have the disease of interest.

(f) Write down the parameter space in terms of θ, ϕ, β and γ. Comment on the appropriateness of the 4 parameter scales for calculating confidence intervals in small and large samples, using your results from parts (d) and (e).

7. Consider the common stroke rate model discussed in Section 4.8.2 in which Y_i, the number of strokes observed in group i, had a $\text{Poisson}(\lambda F_i)$ distribution, where F_i was the number of person-years of observation in group i, for $i = 1, 2$. Now suppose that we adopt a model in which there is an additional number of strokes which has a mean $\theta > 0$ that is independent of the period of observation, so that

$$Y_i \stackrel{d}{=} \text{Poisson}(\theta + \lambda F_i) \qquad i = 1, 2.$$

(a) Write down the log-likelihood associated with this model, $\ell(\lambda, \theta)$.

(b) Differentiate $\ell(\lambda, \theta)$ with respect to λ and θ to obtain the likelihood equations. Do these likelihood equations lead to explicit MLEs for λ and θ?

(c) Write down the sum of squares, $SS(\lambda, \theta) = (y_1 - \mu_1)^2 + (y_2 - \mu_2)^2$, where $\mu_i = E(Y_i)$ and y_i is the observed value of the random variable Y_i.

(d) Differentiate $SS(\lambda, \theta)$ with respect to λ and θ to obtain the least squares estimating equations.

(e) Solve the least squares estimating equations from part (d) to obtain the least squares estimates of λ and θ. Hence obtain least squares estimates $\tilde{\lambda}$ and $\tilde{\theta}$ for the data described in Section 4.8.1.

(f) Write down an advantage and a disadvantage of least squares estimation for this model, compared with maximum likelihood estimation.

8. Consider estimation of the stroke rate ratio γ, as discussed in Section 4.8.4. Suppose that the stroke rate in group 1, λ_1, is a nuisance parameter that we have no interest in.

(a) Using the discussion in Section 3.7.5, write down the profile likelihood as a function of γ alone, $L(\gamma)$, and the profile log-likelihood, $\ell(\gamma)$.

(b) By comparing back to the results in Section 4.8.4, show that the estimate of γ obtained by maximising the profile log-likelihood $\ell(\gamma)$ is the same as the estimate obtained by maximising the full log-likelihood in terms of γ and λ_1.

(c) Using the expected information corresponding to the profile log-likelihood $\ell(\gamma)$, calculate a standard error associated with the estimate from part (b).

(d) Construct a 95% confidence interval for γ on the basis of your results from part (c), and compare it with the confidence interval obtained in Section 4.8.5 based on the full log-likelihood.

9. For each of the following distributions, determine the method of moments estimator of θ and decide whether it is the same as the MLE.

(a) $\text{Bin}(n, \theta)$

(b) $\text{Pois}(\theta)$

(c) $\text{Uniform}(0, \theta)$

5

Hypothesis testing concepts

In Chapter 2 we discussed using confidence intervals to conclude whether or not particular values of the parameter are plausible. This introduced us to the notion of hypothesis testing, the principles of which will be developed in the next two chapters. In this chapter we will discuss some of the basic concepts in hypothesis testing, including significance level, power and P-values, and further discuss the connection between hypothesis testing and confidence intervals. Chapter 6 will then make use of these concepts to develop general methods for carrying out hypothesis tests based on the likelihood function. Our discussion in this chapter and the next will present hypothesis tests as rules for deciding whether an hypothesis should be rejected or not, based on the observed sample. This is useful for assessing the statistical significance of observed departures from the hypothesis, but reliance on a simple dichotomy can often lead to misinterpretation, so we will also discuss the importance of viewing hypothesis testing as complementary to the process of confidence interval estimation. These notions will be illustrated using an extended example involving randomised treatment comparisons.

5.1 Hypotheses

In most biostatistical contexts involving hypothesis testing, one is interested in assessing whether there is evidence that a particular factor has an effect on some health outcome. In practice, the term "effect" is often used loosely to encompass both situations that truly are the assessment of the effect of a factor, such as a randomised trial of an intervention, and situations involving only the assessment of associations, such as an observational study of a particular exposure. In either situation, statistical hypothesis testing begins with the development of a probability model, as was used in our discussions on parameter estimation. However, rather than using the sample to estimate the unknown parameter value, hypothesis testing assesses whether the "no effect" value of the parameter can be rejected because it is implausible based on the observed sample. If it can be rejected, then it is reasonable to conclude that the factor under study does have an "effect" on the outcome of interest. Throughout this chapter we will frame the discussion in terms of hypothesis testing associated with an effect parameter such as a rate ratio or mean difference, however, the discussion applies to any parameter in a probability model.

The basis of hypothesis testing is the specification of a **null hypothesis** (H_0) representing the no effect, or null, value of the unknown parameter in our probability model. An hypothesis test is then a procedure for using the observed sample to decide whether there is sufficient evidence to reject the no effect null hypothesis in favour of an **alternative hypothesis** (H_1) that specifies the existence of an effect. The most common null and alternative hypotheses are of the form

$$H_0 : \theta = \theta_0 \quad \text{versus} \quad H_1 : \theta \neq \theta_0$$

where θ is the unknown parameter and θ_0 denotes the no effect value of the parameter in our model. In this case, the null hypothesis is said to be a **simple hypothesis** since it involves only a single value of the parameter, whereas the alternative hypothesis is said to be a **composite hypothesis** since it involves multiple values of the parameter. In the above case the alternative hypothesis is also referred to as a **two-sided hypothesis**, because it covers values of the parameter on both sides of the null value.

In some cases, information may be available about the type of relationship that could potentially exist between the factor and outcome under study, which would restrict the possible values that the parameter could take if it is not equal to the null value. The most common hypothesis specification of this type is

$$H_0 : \theta = \theta_0 \quad \text{versus} \quad H_1 : \theta > \theta_0.$$

In this case the alternative hypothesis is referred to as a **one-sided hypothesis**, because it covers values of the parameter on only one side of the null value. This type of alternative hypothesis may be of interest when it is reasonable to assume the parameter can take on values only on one side of the null value, as might be the case if it can be assumed that the factor under study can only have either no effect or a positive effect on the outcome of interest. However, this assumption is often difficult to justify, and for this reason two-sided hypotheses are more common in practice.

Both the two-sided and one-sided hypothesis specifications described above involve the testing of a simple null hypothesis corresponding to a single parameter value, versus a composite alternative hypothesis corresponding to a range of parameter values. While this is the most common approach, and will be the approach assumed in this chapter unless stated otherwise, it is possible to specify other types of hypotheses. In principle it is possible to specify simple hypotheses, that is hypotheses involving only one parameter value, for both the null and alternative hypotheses. Such hypotheses would require the specification of a single value θ_1 that the parameter would take in the case that it was not equal to the no effect value θ_0. This leads to hypotheses of the form

$$H_0 : \theta = \theta_0 \quad \text{versus} \quad H_1 : \theta = \theta_0.$$

While such hypotheses are of some importance from a theoretical point of view, they are rarely of any practical interest, since it would rarely be the case that only two possible values of a parameter could hold. An additional type of hypothesis specification is where both null and alternative hypotheses are composite. In this case, rather than a single value specifying no effect, a range of values would correspond to no effect, such as

$$H_0 : \theta \leq \theta_0 \quad \text{versus} \quad H_1 : \theta > \theta_0.$$

Composite null hypotheses involve increased complexity in hypothesis tests, but are of some practical importance. In general, however, the examples that we will consider will focus on the testing of a simple null hypothesis against a composite alternative hypothesis.

5.2 Statistical tests

Having specified null and alternative hypotheses, a statistical test is a procedure, or a rule, for using the observed sample to decide whether or not to reject the null hypothesis in favour of the alternative hypothesis. In previous chapters we introduced certain concepts related to our sample and our model that are useful in providing a precise statement of what a statistical test is. Recall that a statistic is any function $T(Y)$ of the sample Y that does not depend on the parameter θ, while the parameter space consists of all possible values for θ. The specification of our statistical test begins with the choice of a statistic, $T(Y)$, on which the rule for rejecting (or not rejecting) the null hypothesis will be based. In this chapter we will not discuss how to make this choice, but in Chapter 6 we will consider general methods that supply us with an appropriate statistic on which to base our test.

The second stage in the specification of our statistical test is to identify which part, or subset, of the parameter space corresponds to values of the parameter covered by H_0, and which part corresponds to values covered by H_1. These subsets of the parameter space should together cover all possible values of the parameter and be non-overlapping. Labelling the subsets as Θ_0 and Θ_1, respectively, allows us to rewrite our hypotheses in a general form, regardless of whether the hypotheses are simple or composite:

$$H_0 : \theta \in \Theta_0 \quad \text{versus} \quad H_1 : \theta \in \Theta_1.$$

For the common case of a simple null hypothesis, Θ_0 will consist of just one point, θ_0, while a composite alternative hypothesis will consist of either an interval (one-sided tests) or the union of two intervals (two-sided tests). With this specification, our final step is to define the statistical test to be a rule for deciding whether θ is in Θ_0 or Θ_1, depending on the observed value $T(y)$ of the statistic $T(Y)$. We specify this rule by considering all possible values that $T(y)$ could take, and then identifying a subset of these values, labelled C, such that if the observed value of $T(y)$ is in C then we reject the null hypothesis. Our decision rule, or hypothesis testing procedure, can therefore be stated in full as

either reject H_0 if $T(y) \in C$ and conclude $\theta \in \Theta_1$

or accept H_0 if $T(y) \notin C$ and conclude $\theta \in \Theta_0$.

Often hypothesis tests involve a simple null hypothesis versus a two-sided alternative hypothesis, where the collection of values C refers to all values exceeding a certain cut-off c. In this case the decision rule can be stated more simply as

either reject H_0 if $T(y) \geq c$ and conclude $\theta \neq \theta_0$

or accept H_0 if $T(y) < c$ and conclude $\theta = \theta_0$.

On the face of it, this decision rule seems to provide a basis for either discounting or confirming the null hypothesis. In practice, however, the idea of "acceptance" of the null hypothesis is often more appropriately interpreted as "non-rejection". In other words, accepting the null hypothesis usually does not correspond to concluding that it is true, but rather that it is not possible to reject it. This is a very important point and we will discuss it in detail in the next section.

We refer to the statistic $T(Y)$ as the **test statistic**, while the observed value of this statistic, $T(y)$, is referred to as the **observed test statistic**. The collection of values C that will lead us to reject the null hypothesis is referred to as the **critical region**, while the cut-off value c is referred to as the **critical value** of the test. Expressing a test in terms of a critical region allows greater generality than expressing it in terms of a critical value, because the critical region does not necessarily have to correspond to an interval above a certain cut-off. However, the critical regions for many important tests can be conveniently expressed in terms of critical values and we will therefore frame most of our discussion in terms of critical values.

One of the most important aspects of hypothesis testing is to decide what test statistic to use, and having decided on the test statistic, what critical value to use. In the extended example and exercises we will study some specific examples of test statistics without considering how the test statistic is chosen. In Chapter 6, however, we will consider general methods for choosing appropriate test statistics, based on the likelihood function. Having chosen the test statistic, the important decision of what critical region to use is based on the notion of controlling statistical errors, which we will discuss later in the chapter.

5.3 Acceptance versus non-rejection

The above purely theoretical description of an hypothesis test may seem to imply that we will either reject the null hypothesis and accept the alternative hypothesis, or else accept the null hypothesis and reject the alternative hypothesis. In fact, while it will be reasonable to conclude that if the null hypothesis is rejected then the alternative hypothesis must be accepted, the question of what interpretation to draw when the null hypothesis is not rejected is less clear.

From one point of view, it may be argued that in the absence of evidence to the contrary we should assume that no effect exists, and that a failure to reject the null hypothesis leads us to accept the "default" option as true. Thus, if the test statistic was in the critical region we would reject the null hypothesis, and if it was not in the critical region we would accept the null hypothesis. From a practical point of view, however, this can be misinterpreted because in most situations a failure to reject the null hypothesis does not correspond to a confirmation that it is true. In particular, as we shall discuss later in this chapter, although one explanation for a failure to reject the null hypothesis is that the null hypothesis is indeed true, another explanation is that the size of our sample was too small to be confident that the true effect is different from the null value. Almost always in biostatistical applications, a failure to reject the null hypothesis should be interpreted as an inconclusive lack of evidence for an effect, rather than providing conclusive evidence that there is no effect. Thus, we generally do not interpret a statistical test as a rule to decide whether to reject or accept the null hypothesis, but rather a rule to decide whether to reject or not reject the null hypothesis.

The above discussion leads us to the importance of estimation concepts as a complement to information obtained from hypothesis testing. Just as a failure to reject the null hypothesis does not constitute a confirmation that it is true, nor does an acceptance of the alternative hypothesis give us precise information about the unknown value of the parameter. It is for this reason that the simple dichotomy of hypothesis testing needs to be combined with the more detailed information available from estimation, particularly confidence intervals. In particular, when a null hypothesis is rejected, a confidence interval can be used to provide more detailed information about the magnitude of the effect, whereas if the null hypothesis is not rejected, a confidence interval can be used to assess how far away from the null value the true effect could plausibly be.

5.4 Statistical errors

When the above testing procedure is used to decide whether or not to reject the null hypothesis, there is clearly the possibility that the resulting decision will not reflect reality. In practice we would not know whether we had made an incorrect conclusion based on our hypothesis test, just as we would not know whether our confidence interval covers the unknown true value of the parameter. These unidentifiable "errors" can be thought of as falling into two distinct types. The desire to minimise the chance that either one of these errors might occur is an important consideration in choosing the test statistic and critical region of the test.

The two types of possible errors correspond, respectively, to an incorrect conclusion in a circumstance where the null hypothesis is true, and an incorrect conclusion in a circumstance where the alternative hypothesis is true. Thus, the first type of hypothesis testing error, referred to as a **type I error**, corresponds to reaching a decision to reject the null hypothesis when in fact it is true, while the second type of error, referred to as a **type II error**, corresponds to reaching a decision not to reject the null hypothesis when in fact the alternative hypothesis is true. These scenarios are summarised in Table 5.1.

TABLE 5.1

Hypothesis test decisions

	Reject H_0	Do not reject H_0
H_0 is true	Type I error	Correct decision
H_1 is true	Correct decision	Type II error

Since type I and type II errors are clearly undesirable, our goal is to construct statistical tests that control the probabilities of these errors occurring. In practice, there is a trade-off between the chance of a type I error and the chance of a type II error. To consider this we will focus on the situation where the critical region can be defined based on the critical value c of the test statistic. For a given sample size, increasing c (or reducing the critical region) will lead to a decrease in the probability of a type I error α and an increase in the probability of a type II error β. Decreasing c will have the opposite effect of increasing the probability of a type I error and decreasing the probability of a type II error. Thus, it is not possible to simultaneously lower both α and β by altering the critical value c of the test statistic.

In view of this trade-off between type I and type II error probability, the "classical" approach to hypothesis testing is to begin by choosing a critical value for the test statistic so as to achieve a suitably low type I error probability. Often the definition of suitably low is taken to be $\alpha = 0.05$, although this is arbitrary and can in principle be fixed at whatever level is considered appropriate for controlling the chance of rejecting the null hypothesis when it is in fact true. Once this objective has been achieved, attention can be focussed on the type II error, and the test manipulated so as to control β, in ways discussed in the next section. The primary focus on the type I error is consistent with the fact that, while it is important to control both types of error, it is usually more important to control the tendency for incorrectly identifying positive effects, than the tendency for an inconclusive result when an effect actually exists.

The specific approach to choosing a critical value that will achieve the desired type I error probability is as follows. Based on the distribution of the test statistic under the assumption that the null hypothesis is true, the critical value is taken to be the value that the test statistic will exceed with probability α. That is, the critical value c is determined by the equation

$$\Pr\big(T(Y) \geq c \mid \theta = \theta_0\big) = \alpha.$$

The above probability statement uses the notation that we introduced in Chapter 3, which in the present context means the probability of the event $T(Y) \geq c$ under the assumption that $\theta = \theta_0$, that is, under the assumption that H_0 is true. For example, this probability might be determined by a normal distribution with mean $\theta = 0$.

In interpreting the type I error probability it is useful to bear in mind the repeated sampling interpretation of frequentist probability. Based on this interpretation we expect that in repeated studies of an identical nature on a population in which no "effect" exists, a proportion α of these studies will nonetheless conclude that an effect does exist. By choosing α to be low we limit the tendency for this to occur, however, we can never fully exclude it. The fact that we expect a certain proportion of tests to reject the null hypothesis purely on the play of chance, is important for interpreting the results from multiple studies, or multiple tests conducted on the same study. Such multiple testing issues will be considered further in the exercises.

5.5 Power and sample size

In the previous section we discussed how, given a particular test statistic, we can determine the critical value that ensures the type I error probability is controlled at an acceptably low level. Having ensured this, the next question is how to limit the type II error probability to an acceptably low level. As we have already discussed, the error probabilities α and β compete with each other in the sense that lowering α tends to raise β. This property, however, is only true for a fixed sample size. When the study design is such that the sample size is flexible, an increase in the sample size will lead to a decrease in the chance of a type II error. This provides the fundamental approach to controlling the type II error.

An important quantity related to the type II error is the **power** of the test. The power is defined as $1 - \beta$, and corresponds to the probability of rejecting the null hypothesis when the null hypothesis is false. In Table 5.1, the power is represented by the decision cell in the lower left-hand corner and therefore corresponds to a correct decision. Thus, in constructing our test it is desirable to have high power. Since power is just one minus the probability of a type II error, there is a mathematical equivalence between controlling the type II error probability to be acceptably low, and controlling the power to be acceptably high. In practice, however, it is more common to express such considerations in terms of power, particularly in relation to determining the sample size. Common values for the power are 0.9 and 0.8, which are usually referred to as 90% or 80% power, and which correspond to values of 0.1 or 0.2 for β.

In our previous discussion of the critical value that will ensure a desired type I error, our calculations were carried out under the assumption that the null hypothesis was true. This corresponds to making the assumption that the parameter takes a single particular value θ_0. In considering the power of the test we must consider the probability of rejecting the null hypothesis under the assumption that the alternative hypothesis is true. However, the alternative hypothesis does not correspond to a specific parameter value, but rather a range of values. Thus, the power will depend on whatever alternative hypothesis parameter value we choose to consider. This leads to a function of the parameter, which is referred to as the **power function** or **power curve**. This can be expressed as

$$\text{Power}(\theta) = \Pr\big(T(Y) \geq c \mid \theta\big)$$

where the dependence on θ reflects the fact that the distribution of the test statistic will depend on whatever alternative hypothesis value is considered for θ. For example, the test statistic may have a normal distribution with mean θ.

We consider some specific examples of power in the extended example. In general, however, the following two general properties hold for the power of a statistical test:

1. For a particular sample size, the power will increase as the value of θ gets further away from the null value θ_0;

2. For a particular value of θ, the power will increase as the sample size gets larger.

The first property reflects the fact that if the size of the effect is large, then we have greater chance of identifying this effect. The second property reflects the fact that the power can be increased by increasing the sample size, and it is this fact that we use to ensure an adequate power is achieved, as we now describe.

The usual approach is to begin by specifying an effect size such that if this represents the truth then we would want to have high power to reject the null hypothesis of no effect. This effect size will correspond to a particular alternative hypothesis value for the parameter, which we will call θ_1. The power assuming θ_1 is the true parameter value is given above by $\text{Power}(\theta_1)$. If our desired power is $1 - \beta$, then the sample size can be chosen so as to achieve this desired power. In particular, using property 2 above, we can increase the sample size until the desire power is achieved:

$$\text{increase } n \text{ until Power}(\theta_1) \geq 1 - \beta.$$

The effect size used in the power calculations may be interpreted as the smallest effect that is of any practical importance, and is sometimes referred to as the **detectable difference**. The concept of a practically important effect will be illustrated further in the extended example. The idea is to distinguish small effects of little practical importance, from large effects that would be of substantial practical importance if they exist. In considering the power of the study, we would like to ensure adequate power for "detecting" the important effect sizes, but would not be too concerned about the power achieved for effect sizes so small as to be unimportant from a practical point of view. Often there may be doubt about the smallest effect size that is of practical importance, so a number of different values for the detectable difference may be of interest. In this case, power calculations may be conducted under a number of different assumptions for θ_1, to assess the sensitivity of the power (or the required sample size) to different values.

We make note also of one additional complication in considering the power of a study. While there may be a particular parameter θ that we are interested in testing an hypothesis about, in practice our probability model may have other parameters as well. Just as we have to specify the value of θ to carry out a power calculation, so too will we need to specify the value of any other parameters. These values may need to be determined based on data from other studies, or a range of plausible values may be considered based on experience with the context under study. A common example of this is when we are interested in testing an hypothesis about the mean of a normal distribution, and we need to make an assumption about the variance of that distribution to assess the power of the study. The extended example illustrates the need to make assumptions about other parameter values when undertaking power calculations.

Determining the sample size to achieve a desired power is a study design issue that needs to be considered prior to the study beginning, and is useful when the size of the study is flexible. If the sample size is not flexible then the power cannot be manipulated in this way and we will need to hope the power we end up with is acceptably high. If power calculations indicate that this is not the case then the study should perhaps be reconsidered. This avoids wasting resources by conducting a study that has a substantial chance of not concluding that there is evidence of an effect, even when the truth is that an important effect exists.

While the sample size is an important way to increase the power, the choice of test statistic can also have an effect on the power. This is an important topic in theoretical statistics, where much effort has been devoted to considering the types of test statistics that lead to the **most powerful test**. In practice, however, the general methods that will be covered in Chapter 6 provide a practical approach to identifying appropriate test statistics that achieve high power among all possible test statistics in parametric models. While we will not consider the theoretical topic of most powerful tests in any detail here, the exercises provide an illustration of the power obtained by two different test statistics applicable to the same situation.

5.6 *P*-values

When an hypothesis test rejects the null hypothesis, the result is said to be **statistically significant**. This terminology reflects the fact that the observed effect size is never exactly equal to the null value specified by the null hypothesis, and the role of an hypothesis test is to identify whether the observed effect size is significant in the sense that it is large relative to what would be expected on the play of chance. Statistical significance only has a meaning when it is interpreted in the context of the critical value that was used for the test, or equivalently the type I error probability α. For example, the result of an hypothesis test may be statistically significant if we choose $\alpha = 0.05$, but not significant if we choose $\alpha = 0.01$. For this reason the conclusion that a null hypothesis is rejected (or not rejected) must be accompanied by the value of α used to conduct the test, and in this context α is referred to as the **significance level** of the test. Thus, the terms significance level and type I error probability may be used interchangeably.

In practice, there will be a particular value for the significance level such that if α is chosen to be larger than this value then the test will be significant and if α is chosen to be smaller than this value then the test will not be significant. This value is referred to as the ***P*-value** of the test, and corresponds to the smallest significance level such that the test would be statistically significant. When the *P*-value does not exceed the significance level α then the test is statistically significant and we can reject the null hypothesis. Conducting our test by checking whether the P-value is above or below the significance level α is effectively equivalent to the procedure described previously of checking whether the test statistic is below or above the critical value c. However, the magnitude of the P-value yields additional information in that it allows us to quantify the degree of statistical significance. In order to understand what is meant by this quantification, we consider the interpretation of the P-value in more detail.

Consider an observed sample y in which the observed value of the test statistic is $t = T(y)$. Since the P-value is the smallest significance level such that the test would be significant, it corresponds to the significance level of a test conducted with a critical value of t. That is, using our definition of the significance level (or type I error probability)

$$P\text{-value} = \Pr\big(T(Y) \geq t \mid \theta = \theta_0\big).$$

Thus, the P-value represents the probability, under the assumption that the null hypothesis is true ($\theta = \theta_0$), of obtaining a test statistic at least as large as the one we observed. This provides a useful intuitive interpretation for the process of hypothesis testing. In particular, a small P-value corresponds to an observed test statistic that is unlikely under the assumption that the null hypothesis is true. If it is sufficiently unlikely to be as large as the one observed, that is, with probability less than α, then we conclude that the null hypothesis is inconsistent with our observed sample and we will reject it in favour of the alternative hypothesis.

The repeated sampling interpretation of probability is again useful to bear in mind in interpreting the probability statement that defines the P-value. It means that if we were to repeat a large number of identical studies on a population in which there was no effect, then the proportion of studies that yielded a test statistic more extreme than the one we obtained will equal the P-value. Thus, the P-value denotes the proportion of studies that would obtain results as extreme as ours, purely on the play of chance. When this proportion is small, we reject chance as a potential explanation of our results, and conclude that there must be a non-null effect size. Of course, in any particular situation the word "effect" must be interpreted carefully, and for non-randomised studies it will usually mean "association".

In interpreting the magnitude of a P-value it is important to recall our previous discussion on the issue of acceptance and non-rejection of the null hypothesis. While a small P-value is a useful indicator that the null hypothesis is implausible, a large P-value cannot be interpreted as indicating support for the null hypothesis. In particular, it is a serious misinterpretation to view the P-value as the "probability" that the null hypothesis is true. This mistake is similar to the misinterpretation of confidence intervals that we discussed in Chapter 2, as an interval that contains the true parameter with a probability of 0.95. In both cases the probability statements have no meaning in the context of the frequentist view of probability, however, the mistake is more dangerous in the case of P-values. A large P-value may arise because of a type II error, particularly due to a small sample size. To use a large P-value as support for the null hypothesis would not identify studies in which the effect was large, but the P-value was insignificant due to low power. It is for this reason that confidence intervals should always be quoted with P-values to give a range of plausible values for the effect size. Furthermore, as discussed previously, the interpretation of "accepting" the null hypothesis should be that there is no evidence against a null effect, rather than that there is evidence for a null effect.

5.7 Extended example

The objective of this extended example is to illustrate the important concepts of hypothesis testing within a standard context, namely, the comparison of two proportions in a binomial model for response to HIV treatment. As well as demonstrating the basic concepts, such as test statistics, significance level, and P-values, we focus on the appropriate interpretation of results from an hypothesis test, particularly when the null hypothesis is not rejected. In relation to this, we focus on the concept of practical significance, and contrast it with statistical significance. Leading on from this we explore how power is related to detectable difference and sample size, and consider the determination of sample size to achieve the desired power. Finally, we illustrate some additional issues related to hypothesis tests, in particular their relationship with confidence intervals.

5.7.1 Randomised interventions

We consider a study involving individuals who are HIV positive, and consider the comparison of two possible antiviral treatments. The first treatment, which we can interpret as the standard or control therapy, involves using a single drug to reduce the extent of HIV in the body. The second treatment, which we can interpret as the experimental therapy, involves administering the control therapy in combination with a second drug. We will refer to the control treatment as mono-therapy and the experimental treatment as combination therapy. The treatment that each individual receives is determined by **randomisation**, by which we mean that equal numbers of individuals are randomly assigned to each treatment. The goal of the study is to compare the two therapies with respect to the "response" to treatment. The main outcome of treatment is the binary indicator of whether or not viral load is adequately reduced at the end of a six month period of treatment. Thus, the study aims to compare the proportion of patients who achieve an adequate response in each treatment group. We will call these proportions the "response rates". In reality they are not really rates, they are proportions, however this terminology is common in health and medical applications. The central quantity that will be used to compare the response rates is their observed difference, which can be considered an estimate of the difference in population response rates.

We have already discussed earlier in this chapter that there could be two explanations for the magnitude of the observed treatment difference: a genuine therapy effect or simply chance. The role of the P-value is to assess the extent to which chance is a plausible explanation, and if it is not, this would leave only a genuine therapy effect as an explanation of the observed difference. There is, however, a third potential explanation. In practice, it is possible that there could be bias caused by differences between the groups being compared which may lead to an apparent difference between the treatments. This is referred to as **confounding**. In this book we are focussing on the principles of statistical inference under the assumption that our sample is not biased, but in practice it is a very important issue to justify a lack of bias. Randomised studies, in which people are assigned to comparison groups at random, are the best way to avoid confounding in assessing interventions. In particular, they ensure that comparison groups are similar in all respects except the intervention under study, thus eliminating bias as an explanation of differences between treatments. Of course, randomisation is not always feasible or ethical, particularly when we are interested in comparing groups that are not defined by an intervention. In this case, epidemiological or observational studies are often used to study groupings defined by exposures, lifestyles and other characteristics.

5.7.2 Model and hypotheses

A natural model for the data from our randomised trial is the two sample binomial model. Throughout we will subscript quantities associated with the control therapy by a 0 and the combination therapy by a 1. Let n be the total number of individuals in the study, with the number on each therapy being $n_0 = n_1 = n/2$, since the number in each group is equal. The full sample is $y = (y_1, \ldots, y_n)$, where y_i is 1 if individual i responded to treatment and is 0 otherwise. However, this full sample can be reduced to the sufficient statistics x_0 and x_1, the observed numbers achieving a response on the two therapies, respectively. There are two parameters in the model, p_0 and p_1, the population response rates for each therapy. Assuming independence of the outcome from each individual, the model assumes that x_0 and x_1 are the observed values of random variables with $\text{Bin}(n_0, p_0)$ and $\text{Bin}(n_1, p_1)$ distributions, respectively. These parameters are estimated by the sample response rates $\hat{p}_0 = x_0/n$ and $\hat{p}_1 = x_1/n$.

For the purpose of hypothesis testing it makes sense to focus on the response rate difference, $\theta = p_1 - p_0$, which is estimated by the sample response rate difference $\hat{\theta} = \hat{p}_1 - \hat{p}_0$. Then the null value specifying no treatment difference is 0, and a two-sided pair of hypotheses is

$$\text{H}_0 : \theta = 0 \quad \text{versus} \quad \text{H}_1 : \theta \neq 0.$$

While this is a natural way to express the treatment difference it is not the only way. For example, we could have used the ratio of the response rates with a null value of 1. Note that the two-sided alternative hypothesis specifies a difference either in favour of the combination therapy ($\theta > 0$) or in favour of the mono-therapy ($\theta < 0$). It may be possible to argue for a one-sided alternative hypothesis $\text{H}_1 : \theta > 0$, if it could be argued that adding an additional therapy could only improve the response rate. However, this will usually be a difficult argument to make. For example, in our case it would seem plausible that extra toxicities from the more intensive combination therapy could potentially lead to less effectiveness than the mono-therapy. Thus, it

TABLE 5.2

Observed data for a randomised study of HIV therapies

	Mono-therapy	Combination therapy	Total
Response	$x_0 = 47$	$x_1 = 57$	104
No response	53	43	96
Total	$n_0 = 100$	$n_1 = 100$	$n = 200$

would seem sensible to allow for both alternatives, and this will usually be the case in biostatistical applications.

5.7.3 Testing for a difference

The data can be summarised in a cross-tabulation that can be analysed using a comparison of proportions test or χ^2 test. We discuss the construction of the associated test statistics based on the observed data in Table 5.2.

Based on these data the estimated response rates are $\hat{p}_0 = 0.47$ and $\hat{p}_1 = 0.57$, with a response rate difference of $\hat{\theta} = 0.10$ in favour of the combination therapy. One approach to constructing a test statistic is based on the distribution of the estimator of the treatment difference assuming the null hypothesis is true. It is necessary to consider this distribution under the assumption that the null hypothesis is true, because the critical value for our test statistic is determined based on this distribution. In the present situation the estimate $\hat{\theta}$ is an observation from an approximate normal distribution, using the normal approximation to the binomial distribution. Assuming the null hypothesis to be true, the population response rates in the two therapy groups are equal, $p_0 = p_1 = p$, and the normal distribution has mean $\theta = 0$, with variance $4p(1-p)/n$. Based on the observed data, and assuming the null hypothesis to be true, our best estimate of the common response rate p is $\hat{p} = 104/200 = 0.52$, leading to an approximate normal distribution of $N(0, 0.0707^2)$ for the estimator of the treatment difference, under the assumption that the null hypothesis is true. Thus, the standardised quantity

$$z = \frac{\hat{\theta}}{\sqrt{4\hat{p}(1-\hat{p})/n}} = 1.415$$

is an observation from a random variable Z with an approximate standard normal distribution, assuming the null hypothesis is true.

Based on the two-sided alternative hypothesis, large positive or large negative values of $\hat{\theta}$ indicate departures from the null hypothesis. This suggests two possible test statistics that we will know the distributions of under the null hypothesis, namely, $t_1 = |z|$ and $t_2 = z^2$ which are the observed values of random variables $T_1 = |Z|$ and $T_2 = Z^2$.

The critical values for these test statistics, c_1 and c_2, are determined by

$$\Pr(T_1 \geq c_1 \mid \theta = 0) = \Pr(|Z| \geq c_1 \mid \theta = 0) = \alpha$$

and

$$\Pr\left(T_2 \geq c_2 \mid \theta = 0\right) = \Pr\left(Z^2 \geq c_2 \mid \theta = 0\right) = \alpha.$$

Here, the probability refers to the standard normal distribution of Z, assuming the null hypothesis is true. Thus, using a conventional significance level of $\alpha = 0.05$, and using the fact that the square of a standard normal random variable is a $\chi^2(1)$ random variable, we obtain critical values of 1.96 and 3.84 for the two test statistics, respectively.

Not surprisingly, we can see that the two approaches will give equivalent results, since $1.96^2 = 3.84$. The second approach can be shown to equivalent to a χ^2 test for independence. That is, conducting a χ^2 test for a 2×2 table is equivalent to conducting a two-sided comparison of two binomial proportions, and it therefore does not matter which one we use. For our observed data set, since $z^2 = 1.415^2 = 2.00 < 3.84$, our test is not statistically significant and we would therefore not reject the null hypothesis that the response rate on combination therapy equals the response rate on mono-therapy.

According to our definition of the P-value, which we will just call P,

$$P = \Pr\left(T_2 \geq t_2 \mid \theta = 0\right) = \Pr\left(Z^2 \geq 2.00 \mid \theta = 0\right) = \mathbf{0.16} > \alpha = 0.05.$$

Thus, we would not reject the null hypothesis on the basis of the P-value, which is consistent with the result obtained by comparing the test statistic with the critical value. However, the P-value allows us to quantify how extreme our result is, relative to what we could have expected purely on the play of chance. Indeed, it is useful to think of the repeated sampling framework and imagine a large number of identical randomised trials, conducted on a population that has equal response rates for the two therapies. Figure 5.1 plots the observed value of the test statistic T_1 for 1000 such studies, simulated based on the assumption that there is no difference in response rates between the two therapies. Given where the observed test statistic from our sample lands on this plot, with approximately $P = 16\%$ of the studies exceeding the value 2.0, it is quite plausible that our test statistic could have arisen from a population that has identical response rates for the two therapies. This explains why we would not be in a position to reject the null hypothesis of equal response rates based on our data. Notice, however, that with a more extreme hypothetical test statistic of say 8.0, it would be somewhat implausible that such a value arose from such a population, and it would therefore be reasonable to reject the hypothesis of equal response rates.

5.7.4 Interpretation

In view of the insignificant result obtained above, it is useful to return to our discussion of the difference between acceptance and non-rejection of the null hypothesis. Previously we argued that a failure to reject the null hypothesis should be interpreted as an inconclusive result, rather than evidence that the null hypothesis is true. A confidence interval for the response rate difference is useful for illustrating this. Based on the standard errors for each of the response rates, a standard error for the response

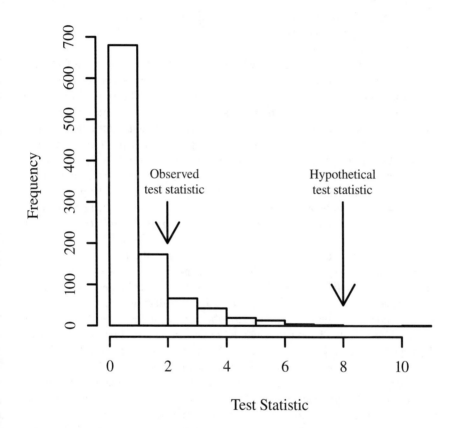

FIGURE 5.1

Histogram of test statistics (T_2) from 1000 studies on a population with no difference in response rates between therapies

rate difference is

$$\mathrm{se}(\hat{\theta}) = \sqrt{\hat{p}_0(1-\hat{p}_0)/100 + \hat{p}_1(1-\hat{p}_1)/100} = 0.0703.$$

Thus, a 95% confidence interval is $0.10 \pm 1.96 \times 0.0703 = (-0.04, 0.24)$, for the true response rate difference between the two therapies. The range of this confidence interval shows that, although we do not have evidence that there is a non-null effect, we cannot rule out an effect size as large as 24% in favour of the combination therapy. That is, we cannot rule out a 24% greater response rate on combination therapy, in absolute terms. This confidence interval shows that if we consider such an effect as large, then we are not in a position to accept the null hypothesis, despite having been unable to reject the null hypothesis.

It is useful at this point to consider what we would define as a "large" effect. This is a clinical question rather than a statistical question, and depends on the magnitude of effect that would be considered of practical significance. The notion of practical significance will depend very much on the situation, but in this context it might be considered to be the magnitude of effect that would lead clinicians to change clinical practice and adopt the new combination therapy as the standard of care. Suppose in our situation a 10% larger response rate on the combination therapy would be required to change clinical practice. This would mean that, when compared to the control therapy, one extra viral load response is achieved for each 10 patients that are treated with the combination therapy. By comparing our confidence interval with this practically significant effect, it is clear that we can neither rule out effects of an important magnitude nor effects of an unimportant magnitude. This is consistent with the inconclusive result that we obtained from the hypothesis test.

It is instructive to consider a number of other potential results that could have arisen, along with their *P*-values, to get a feel for the distinction between practical significance and statistical significance. Figure 5.2 considers such results, beginning with the confidence interval for the data described above, and followed by four other confidence intervals that hypothetically might have arisen. The first two alternative results depict statistically significant situations in which it would be reasonable to conclude that the response rates favour the combination therapy group. However, notice that only in the first case would it be reasonable to strongly conclude that the effect is of practical significance, since the second result could not exclude response rate differences between 0 and 10%. The third alternative result is potentially misleading because the statistical significance may appear to suggest that there is an important advantage of combination therapy over mono-therapy. However, the magnitude of this response rate difference is of a magnitude that would not be considered of any practical significance, and has likely arisen because of a very large sample size. This shows that statistical significance does not necessarily imply practical significance, particularly if a very large sample size is used in a situation where the effect is minimal. The final alternative result is not statistically significant as in our original analysis, however, it differs in that it excludes all response rate differences of a magnitude that are of any practical significance. Thus, if ever we were prepared to "accept" the null hypothesis, this would be such a situation since it is reasonable to exclude the possibility of a practically significant effect. In general, however, it

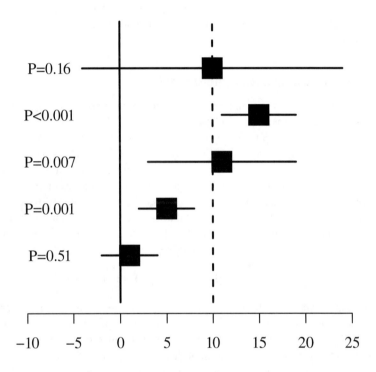

Treatment Difference (%) and 95% CI

FIGURE 5.2
Treatment difference estimates and 95% confidence intervals for the observed data (top line) and four hypothetical data sets. The dashed line denotes the practically significant treatment effect (10%)

is wise to limit such acceptance to situations where the study has been specifically designed to confirm the equivalence of two treatments, using a special design called an **equivalence study**. One reason for this is that opportunistic post hoc choice of the practically important difference could be used to inappropriately argue that the two treatments are equivalent. Equivalence studies are beyond our scope in this book, but an introduction is provided in Armitage et al. (2002) together with discussion of a number of other special types of randomised clinical trial designs. Overall though, the examples presented in Figure 5.2 illustrate the importance of augmenting an hypothesis test with both a confidence interval and a quantification of the practically important effect size. It is seen that for an effect to be meaningful it should be both practically significant and statistically significant, and that these two concepts are not identical.

5.7.5   Assessing power and sample size

The above analysis was unable to reject the null hypothesis despite the magnitude of the observed treatment difference being identical to the magnitude that we would consider practically significant (10%). We now take a step back to the design stage of this randomised trial, and investigate this issue in relation to power and sample size.

Suppose we were designing the above study and planned to have 200 individuals in the study, 100 on each of the mono and combination therapies. What power would we have for detecting a practically significant treatment difference of 10%? In other words, what is the probability that we will conclude that there is statistically significant evidence of a treatment effect, if the true population treatment difference is 10%? According to our definition of power,

$$\text{Power}(0.1) = \Pr\left(T_1 \geq 1.96 \mid \theta = 0.1\right).$$

Previously we used the distribution of T_1 assuming the null hypothesis was true ($\theta = 0$), however, in order to calculate the above power we need to know the distribution assuming $\theta = 0.1$. An important difference between these two situations is that the variance of the treatment difference estimator is different under the null and alternative hypotheses. This is not always the case, but it introduces an extra level of complexity in the present context. As used above, under the null hypothesis the variance is $V_0/n = 4p(1-p)/n$ where p is the common overall response rate. Under the alternative hypothesis, where the response rates differ, this variance is $V_1/n = \frac{2}{n}\left[p_0(1-p_0) + p_1(1-p_1)\right]$. This implies that the test statistic T_1 is the absolute value of a random variable with the normal distribution

$$N\left(\frac{\theta}{\sqrt{V_0/n}}, \frac{V_1}{V_0}\right).$$

If the variance of the treatment difference estimator was identical under the null and alternative hypotheses, then we would have the simpler situation of a variance equal to 1. It is left as an exercise to verify that the variance is the ratio specified above.

Based on the normal distribution identified above, it is possible to carry out the required power calculation. Notice, however, that although we have specified a value for the treatment difference θ, the power calculation also depends on the parameter values p_0 and p_1, since the distribution of the test statistic depends on these values. These are clearly unknown, however, usually there would be prior information available about the response rate for the control treatment in a randomised trial. Suppose then that we have information from previous studies that suggest a control response rate on the order of 50%. Then, together with our assumption about θ for the power calculation, this would imply that $p_1 = 0.5 + 0.1 = 0.6$. Given the equal sample sizes, the overall response rate would be the average of p_0 and p_1, so that $p = 0.55$. Substituting these values into our normal distribution, we now know that our test statistic T_1 is the absolute value of a $N(1.42, 0.99)$ random variable. Thus, the power of our test with a detectable difference of 10%, is

$$\text{Power}(0.1) = 1 - \Phi\left(\frac{1.96 - 1.42}{\sqrt{0.99}}\right) + \Phi\left(\frac{-1.96 - 1.42}{\sqrt{0.99}}\right) = 0.29$$

where Φ is the standard normal cumulative distribution function. A power on the order of 29% would be considered very low, and it is generally more appropriate to have a power on the order of 80–90%. In particular, with an approximately 70% chance of not finding a significant difference even if the true difference was 10%, it is perhaps not surprising that the study with 200 individuals did not conclude that there was a statistically significant difference between the response rates on the two therapies.

We can carry out the same calculations for values of θ other than 0.1. A plot of the resulting power calculations over a range of values for the true treatment difference is provided in Figure 5.3, for a number of different sample sizes. These functions are referred to as power functions or power curves.

Observe that these power functions satisfy the two properties that we highlighted earlier in this chapter: for a fixed sample size the power increases as the treatment difference gets further away from the null, and for a fixed treatment difference the power increases as the sample size increases. It can be seen that if we increase the sample size sufficiently then we will be able to achieve a high power for detecting a treatment difference of 10%. For example, with $n = 1037$ individuals overall the resulting power is 90%. For very small treatment differences it can be seen that the power is very low, however, this would not concern us because such treatment differences are of little practical significance. All power curves have the value 5% at $\theta = 0$ because this corresponds to the null hypothesis, in which case we have $\alpha = 0.05$ for all sample sizes.

Sample size calculation can be carried out by trial and error based on the power function, by trying different sample sizes and calculating the resulting power. When the alternative hypothesis is one-sided it is possible to straightforwardly invert the relationship between power and sample size to give the following formula for the required sample size:

$$n = \frac{1}{\theta^2}\left(z_{1-\alpha}\sqrt{V_0} + z_{1-\beta}\sqrt{V_1}\right)^2.$$

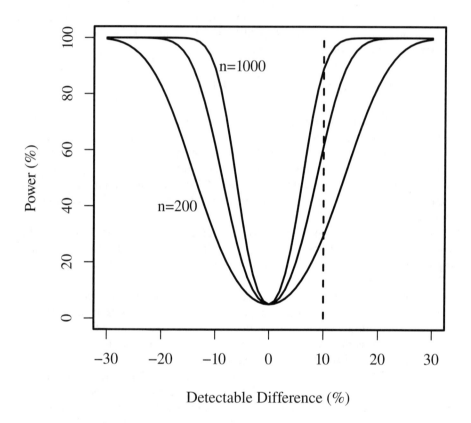

FIGURE 5.3
Power functions for sample sizes of 200, 500 and 1000. The dashed line denotes the practically significant treatment effect (10%)

For two-sided alternative hypotheses, an approximation is to use this formula substituting $\alpha/2$ for α, or else more complex methods can be used based on the χ^2 distribution. The approximate method leads to $n = 1035$ for 90% power in our example, which is in excellent agreement with the calculation of $n = 1037$ obtained above.

5.7.6 Confidence intervals and hypothesis tests

We have already emphasised the importance of augmenting information obtained from hypothesis testing with information obtained from estimation, particularly confidence intervals. In fact there is a correspondence between hypothesis testing and confidence interval estimation. A null hypothesis $H_0 : \theta = \theta_0$ can be tested against a two-sided alternative hypothesis, using a significance level α, by determining whether the value θ_0 is contained in the $100(1 - \alpha)\%$ confidence interval for θ. This is consistent with the intuitive interpretation of a confidence interval as the range of plausible parameter values. Figure 5.2 provides an illustration, where we see that the confidence intervals that do not cover 0 are associated with significant P-values. Figure 5.2 also illustrates how the confidence interval can be used to test the hypothesis that the parameter is equal to any other specific value. For example, in our previous discussions of whether the confidence interval included the practically significant value of 10%, we were effectively carrying out a test of whether we could reject the hypothesis that the true difference is 10%.

Since there is an equivalence between hypothesis testing and confidence interval estimation some statisticians argue that only confidence intervals should be used, because they are less open to misinterpretation than P-values. Nonetheless, the P-value does provide information that a 95% confidence interval does not provide, namely, it quantifies how extreme the results are relative to what could be expected by chance alone. In general, a properly interpreted hypothesis test augmented by a confidence interval provides a more complete summary of the available information.

Another way of looking at the equivalence between confidence intervals and hypothesis tests is that the confidence interval includes any parameter value θ_0 for which we would not reject the null hypothesis $H_0 : \theta = \theta_0$ against a two-sided alternative hypothesis. This fact can be exploited to construct confidence intervals in complicated situations, based on the types of test statistics we will cover in the next chapter.

Exercises

1. In the extended example we discussed a setting in which antiviral drugs were used to reduce HIV viral load, with the binary outcome being whether or not patients achieved adequate suppression of the virus. In these exercises we look at the magnitude of reduction in viral load as a continuous outcome, that is, the

change from just prior to therapy to that achieved after six months of therapy. To simplify things we will just look at the reduction in one of the treatment groups, say the combination therapy group, and consider hypothesis testing of whether the reduction on this therapy is statistically significant. In practice, it would be worthwhile comparing this reduction with that of the control group in a randomised trial. Testing of this type, which is analogous to the two-sample comparisons of proportions in the extended example, will be considered as one of the illustrations in the next chapter. Consider a sample $y = (y_1, \ldots, y_n)$ corresponding to observation of the reduction in viral load over a six month period for n individuals on combination therapy. In this exercise we will assume that this change has a $N(\mu, \sigma^2)$ distribution. We will study the one-sample t-test, which is based on the decision rule

$$\text{reject } H_0 \text{ if } |t| \geq c \qquad \text{where } t = \left| \frac{\bar{y}}{s_{n-1}/\sqrt{n}} \right|$$

and where the test statistic t is an observation from a t_{n-1} distribution if H_0 is true.

(a) Write down the null-hypothesis and two-sided alternative hypothesis that would be of interest for this one-sample context.

(b) Describe how to determine the critical value c for the one-sample t-test, based on a significance level $\alpha = 0.05$, and calculate c for $n = 50$.

(c) Describe how to calculate the P-value for the sample, and calculate it supposing that the mean reduction in viral load was $\bar{y} = 0.2$ and the observed variance was $s_{n-1}^2 = 1.04$.

(d) What would you conclude regarding the hypotheses from part (a)?

(e) Calculate a 95% confidence interval for the mean reduction in viral load μ. Explain how it is consistent with the result in part (d).

(f) Suppose that the reduction in viral load is only of practical benefit if it exceeds 0.3. Interpret this information in the context of your answers to parts (d) and (e).

2. This question concerns the significance level or type I error of the t-test compared to a second test. The second test is called the Wilcoxon signed-rank test, which is a non-parametric test that uses only the ranks of the observations in the sample and not their numerical value. For now, we do not need to define the Wilcoxon signed-rank test in detail but we will discuss it further in Chapter 8. Use the function cnorm.sim described in Appendix 2 to simulate 1000 repeated studies of size 50, from a population in which there is no average reduction in viral load from the treatment. Assume that the variance of the reduction between individuals is 1.0 (on the scale used to measure viral load), and that the reductions are normally distributed.

(a) Write down the interpretation of the significance level of an hypothesis test, in the context of conducting repeated studies.

(b) For each study decide whether the null hypothesis would be rejected or not at the 5% significance level, based on the results of each of the two types of hypothesis tests. Hence obtain a simulation-based estimate of the significance level for each of the two tests.

(c) Based on the results in part (b), do the two tests seem to have the significance level that you would expect?

3. This question concerns the power of the two tests studied in Exercise 2. Use the same assumptions as Exercise 2, except we will now assume that the population does have a reduction in viral load when treated with this therapy.

(a) Write down the interpretation of the power of an hypothesis test, in the context of conducting repeated studies.

(b) Repeat the simulations carried out in Exercise 2, except now assume that the population mean reduction is 0.2, 0.4, 0.6, 0.8 and 1.0 (i.e. carry out 5 additional sets of simulations). For each study decide whether the null hypothesis would be rejected or not at the 5% significance level, based on the results of each of the two types of hypothesis tests. For each value of the mean reduction, obtain a simulation-based estimate of the power for each test.

(c) For a mean reduction ranging from 0 to 1, plot a simulation-based estimate of the power function for each test (plot both functions on the same graph).

(d) What advantage does the t-test have? Based on your simulation results, is it an important advantage and why do you think it arises?

4. Repeat the simulations in Exercises 2 and 3, except use simulation from a "contaminated" normal distribution, in which 90% of observations come from a normal distribution, and 10% of observations are from a distribution that is uniformly distributed between -5 and 5 (i.e. we have a large proportion of outliers in the sample).

(a) Plot the same simulation-based estimates of the power functions for each test, as was carried out in Exercise 3.

(b) Which test seems to have an advantage? Hence summarise the relative merits of each of these tests.

5. Suppose we have a population in which there is no reduction in viral load on average. Suppose we conduct k studies on this population and test whether there is a statistically significant reduction in each case. The test statistic that we use is unimportant for this exercise.

(a) Write down an expression for the probability that at least one of these studies yields a result that is statistically significant, using a significance level of α for each test.

(b) Calculate this for $\alpha = 0.05$, and $k = 1, 2, 3, 5, 10, 15, 20$.

(c) By referring to your results in part (b), summarise the problem with conducting multiple tests and concluding statistical significance if one of them rejects the null hypothesis.

(d) Suppose we let our significance level depend on the number of tests we are conducting. In particular, if we are conducting k tests, suppose we use a significance level of α/k for each test, where $\alpha = 0.05$. Based on this, repeat the calculation in part (b), of the probability that at least one of the studies will yield a statistically significant result.

(e) Using the results of part (d), explain how this correction to the significance level rectifies the problem identified in part (c). (This is called Bonferroni correction for multiple comparisons, which is one of a number of possible approaches to deal with the problem.)

6. Suppose you can approximate the t-distribution by the normal distribution (i.e. assume n is large). Analogous to the expression given in the extended example, the expression for the sample size required for a one-sided test is:

$$n = \frac{\sigma^2}{d^2}(z_{1-\alpha} + z_{1-\beta})^2$$

where d is the detectable difference in the mean viral load reduction. How does the required sample size change as the following quantities increase (give reasons):

(a) The variance of the reduction in viral load?

(b) The detectable difference d?

(c) The power $1 - \beta$?

(d) Justify the above formula.

7. Consider the relationship between power and sample size in Exercise 6. For this question we will assume a one-sided test. Suppose that it is known from prior data that the variance σ^2 is approximately 1.0 and suppose that the hypothesis test will be conducted using a significance level of 5%.

(a) How many patients are required in the study if a power of 80% is desired and the mean viral load reduction is 0.25?

(b) Write down an expression for the power, in terms of the sample size and the detectable difference. Assuming 100 patients are available for the study, what power is achieved if the mean viral load reduction is 0.25?

(c) Write down an expression for the detectable difference, in terms of the sample size and the power. Assuming 100 patients are available for the study, what difference can be detected with a power of 80%?

(d) Suppose that it is anticipated that $D\%$ of patients will not adhere to the therapy. Suppose also that the mean viral load reduction is d in patients who do adhere to therapy, and is 0 in patients who do not adhere to therapy.

What is the mean viral load reduction in a population in which $D\%$ of patients do not adhere to therapy?

(e) Hence write down an expression for the sample size as a function of the desired power, the mean viral load difference d, and the proportion of patients who do not adhere to therapy D.

(f) By what factor would you inflate the sample size in part (a), to account for an expected 10% of patients not adhering to therapy?

6

Hypothesis testing methods

In Chapter 5 we studied general properties of hypothesis tests and illustrated the main concepts using particular examples of hypothesis tests. However, we did not discuss how such tests might be motivated in the first place. Just as we were able to provide a general likelihood-based method for motivating estimators in Chapter 4, so too are we able to provide general likelihood-based methods for motivating hypothesis tests. The objective of this chapter is to present three such methods that can be used in most situations where inference is based on a likelihood function. We begin by presenting the motivation for these methods and describing them in detail when the model involves a single parameter. After comparing the different approaches, we then consider how they extend to situations where the model involves multiple parameters. We will discuss a number of types of hypotheses in multiple parameter situations, particularly the context of testing whether a model can be reduced to a simpler model having a smaller number of parameters. Finally we return to the connection between confidence intervals and hypothesis tests, and its relation to the methods introduced in this chapter. The methods are illustrated using mortality comparisons within a randomised clinical trial.

6.1 Approaches to hypothesis testing

The likelihood function that was used previously as the basis for estimation of unknown parameters can also be used as the basis for testing hypotheses about these parameters. There are three common approaches to making use of the likelihood function for testing hypotheses, and each leads to a general method that can be applied regardless of the statistical model that has been assumed for the sample. The three methods differ in that they are each based on different aspects of the likelihood function: the log-likelihood; the derivative of the log-likelihood (the score function); and the value at which the maximum likelihood is achieved (the MLE). In this chapter we will present each of these methods in detail and discuss their relative merits.

Our discussion of hypothesis testing methods will focus primarily on testing a simple null hypothesis against a two-sided alternative hypothesis. This is a common scenario in biostatistics because we often wish to decide whether to reject the hypothesis that an intervention, risk factor or some other "effect" is unrelated to an outcome of interest. That is, if our parameter θ measures the effect size, and the value θ_0 corresponds to there being no effect, then we are often interested in deciding whether to reject the null hypothesis $\theta = \theta_0$ in favour of the two-sided alternative $\theta \neq \theta_0$. As discussed in Chapter 5, occasionally there are other hypotheses of interest, such as a one-sided alternative or a composite null hypothesis, but the two-sided situation is most common.

Accordingly, our discussion in this chapter will assume, with a few signposted exceptions, that the null and alternative hypotheses are of the form

$$H_0 : \theta = \theta_0 \quad \text{versus} \quad H_1 : \theta \neq \theta_0.$$

We will begin by focussing on models with a single parameter, in other words where θ is one-dimensional, but in later sections we will show how the general methods of hypothesis testing extend naturally to include multiple parameter models.

Before considering the general approaches to hypothesis testing in detail, we start by discussing the idea of measuring the extent to which the sample departs from the null hypothesis. Since the object of our inference is the unknown model parameter, the extent to which the sample departs from the null hypothesis can be measured by the difference between the parameter value under the null hypothesis and the parameter value most supported by the sample. This difference corresponds to the difference between θ_0 and the MLE, $\hat{\theta}$. If this difference is "large" then the sample is inconsistent with the null hypothesis, suggesting we should reject the null hypothesis. We can therefore use this difference as a basis for constructing a test statistic, and hence an hypothesis test.

This leads to the notion of testing our hypotheses using a measure of the difference between the null hypothesis and the sample, $D(\theta_0, \hat{\theta})$, and raises the question: what choices for D are appropriate for measuring the departure of the sample from the null hypothesis? Clearly this difference measure should achieve a minimum of zero when the null hypothesis and the sample coincide, that is when $\hat{\theta} = \theta_0$, and should become increasingly large as the sample departs further from the null hypothesis. With these basic requirements there are many possible choices for D, but there are three in particular that form the basis of the three most common approaches to hypothesis testing. These three choices are based on the log-likelihood function $\ell(\theta) = \log L(\theta)$, the score function $S(\theta) = \ell'(\theta)$, and the simple difference between θ_0 and $\hat{\theta}$:

1. **Log-likelihood difference**: difference between the maximum value of the log-likelihood and the value of the log-likelihood evaluated at the null parameter value

$$D_1(\theta_0, \hat{\theta}) = \ell(\hat{\theta}) - \ell(\theta_0);$$

2. **Score difference**: difference between the value of the log-likelihood derivative or score function, evaluated at the MLE, and the value of the score function evaluated at the null parameter value

$$D_2(\theta_0, \hat{\theta}) = |S(\hat{\theta}) - S(\theta_0)|;$$

3. **Estimate difference**: difference between the MLE and the null parameter value

$$D_3\left(\theta_0, \hat{\theta}\right) = \left|\hat{\theta} - \theta_0\right|.$$

Notice that because $S\left(\hat{\theta}\right) = 0$ by the definition of the MLE, the score "difference" simplifies to $\left|S\left(\theta_0\right)\right|$, and so has the advantage of not requiring calculation of the MLE. Notice also that since $\ell\left(\hat{\theta}\right) \geq \ell\left(\theta_0\right)$ by definition of the MLE, no absolute value signs are necessary in the definition of D_1. More detailed comparison of the three approaches will be considered later in this chapter, after we describe the corresponding hypothesis tests in detail.

We have said that a "large" value for the difference measure indicates that the observed sample is inconsistent with the null hypothesis. However, this is too vague to allow us to actually reject the null hypothesis because we have not specified exactly what is meant by "large". In order to do this, we will need to identify the sampling distribution of each of the difference measures, assuming the null hypothesis is true. This distribution can then be used to define what we mean by an extreme value for our difference measure, and hence to determine the critical value of an hypothesis test. As we will see later, one of the reasons why these three choices are so commonly used in practice is that they all have simple sampling distributions when the sample size is sufficiently large and the difference measure has been appropriately scaled. In the coming sections we will consider this for each of the three approaches. Importantly, these approaches apply to virtually all situations where a likelihood function is available, and can therefore be used regardless of the statistical model that has been assumed for the sample.

6.2   Likelihood ratio test

In Chapter 3 we discussed the likelihood ratio as a measure of the difference in support that the sample has for two parameter values. The log-likelihood difference can be used in the same way, since it is simply the log of a likelihood ratio. This means that the first of our difference measures can be thought of as measuring the difference in support that the sample has for the MLE value as compared to the null parameter value. If this difference is large, then the sample does not provide support for the null hypothesis value. This gives the log-likelihood difference an appealing interpretation and makes it a natural basis for the development of an hypothesis test. The resulting test is referred to as the **likelihood ratio test**, since log-likelihood differences have a one-to-one correspondence with likelihood ratios.

In order to specify the details of the likelihood ratio test we need to understand the sampling distribution of the log-likelihood difference. Of course, we could equivalently try to understand the sampling distribution of the likelihood ratio, but it turns out to be mathematically easier to work on the log scale. The exact distribution of the log-likelihood difference is generally complicated and would only be useful for determining the critical value of a test in a limited number of simple situations. However, when the sample size n is large, then under very general assumptions about the probability model, the sampling distribution has a simple form when the null hypothesis is true. In particular, when the parameter θ is one-dimensional, the observed statistic

$$t_{LR} = 2D_1\left(\theta_0, \hat{\theta}\right) = 2\left[\ell(\hat{\theta}) - \ell(\theta_0)\right] = 2\log\left(\frac{L(\hat{\theta})}{L(\theta_0)}\right)$$

is the observed value of a random variable T_{LR} that has an approximate $\chi^2(1)$ distribution when the null hypothesis is true. Since the non-negative quantity t_{LR} will be large when the sample does not provide support for the null hypothesis value, this leads to a general hypothesis test with significance level α, which is applicable when n is large and there is just one parameter:

Likelihood ratio test :   reject H_0 if $t_{LR} \geq \chi^2_{1-\alpha}(1)$.

Here, the critical value $c = \chi^2_{1-\alpha}(1)$ is the $1 - \alpha$ percentile of the χ^2 distribution with 1 degree of freedom. Since

$$\Pr\left(\text{reject } H_0 \mid \theta = \theta_0\right) = \Pr\left(T_{LR} \geq \chi^2_{1-\alpha}(1) \mid \theta = \theta_0\right) = \alpha,$$

it can be seen that the critical value has been chosen so as to give the likelihood ratio test a significance level α. For example, when using the 5% significance level the critical value is $c = 3.84$.

The theory justifying the asymptotic distribution of the likelihood ratio test statistic, and hence the validity of the above likelihood ratio test, will not be considered in detail here. It is based on a series expansion of the log-likelihood function and will be touched on later in this chapter when we consider the relationship between the various test statistics. An important point in relation to this theory, and the results to follow in relation to the other test statistics, is that they do depend on certain assumptions over and above the large sample size. We will briefly consider some of the more important assumptions later in the chapter, which essentially parallel the caveats identified in Chapter 4, for the asymptotic properties of the MLE. It is worth remembering, however, that these assumptions will be satisfied in the vast majority of situations that are likely to be encountered in practice.

Example 6.1 Consider the stroke incidence study discussed in the extended examples of Chapters 3 and 4. In this example we will assume that the stroke rates in the two diet groups are identical, so that we have a one parameter model. Our data consist of 484 strokes from among 2000 individuals, who were observed for a total of $F = 9805$ person-years. The number of strokes is assumed to follow a Poisson distribution with mean λF, where λ is the stroke rate per person per year. Suppose our goal is to test

$$H_0 : \lambda = 0.05   \text{versus}   H_1 : \lambda \neq 0.05.$$

The log-likelihood function for this sample is $\ell(\lambda) = 484\log(\lambda) - 9805\lambda$ with the corresponding MLE being $\hat{\lambda} = 484/9805 = 0.0494$. The likelihood ratio test statistic is therefore

$$t_{LR} = 2\left[\ell(0.0494) - \ell(0.05)\right] = 0.080.$$

Comparing t_{LR} with the critical value $\chi^2_{0.95}(1) = 3.84$ means that we would not reject the null hypothesis at the 5% significance level, with $P = \Pr\left(\chi^2(1) \geq 0.080\right) = 0.78$.

6.3   Score test

The second test that we consider is based on the second of our difference measures, the score function $S(\theta) = \ell'(\theta)$, evaluated at the null parameter value. The test that comes from using this quantity is referred to as the **score test**. In order to specify such a test, we need to understand the sampling distribution of the score function when it is evaluated at the null hypothesis value. Assuming the null hypothesis is true, it turns out that $S(\theta_0)$ is an observation from a distribution that is approximately normally distributed when the sample size n is large. This normal distribution is $N(0, I(\theta_0))$, where $I(\theta_0)$ is the expected information evaluated at the null hypothesis parameter value. This approximate normality means that when there is just one parameter, the observed statistic

$$t_S = \frac{D_2(\theta_0, \hat{\theta})^2}{I(\theta_0)} = \frac{S(\theta_0)^2}{I(\theta_0)}$$

is the observed value of a random variable T_S that has an approximate $\chi^2(1)$ distribution when the null hypothesis is true. This statement of course makes use of the fact that the square of a standard normal random variable has a $\chi^2(1)$ distribution. The non-negative quantity t_S is interpreted similarly to t_{LR}, in that large values indicate that the sample is inconsistent with the null hypothesis. This again motivates a general hypothesis test applicable when n is large and there is just one parameter:

Score test :   reject H_0 if $t_S \geq \chi^2_{1-\alpha}(1)$.

This test will have significance level α, as described for the likelihood ratio test in the previous section.

Example 6.2 Continuing from Example 6.1, the score function is $S(\lambda) = 484/\lambda - 9805$ and the information is $I(\lambda) = 484/\lambda^2$. The score test statistic is therefore

$$t_S = \frac{S(0.05)^2}{I(0.05)} = 0.081.$$

Since this is less than $\chi^2_{0.95}(1) = 3.84$ we would not reject the null hypothesis at the 5% significance level, and $P = 0.78$. These results are similar, although not identical, to the results from the likelihood ratio test in Example 6.1.

6.4   Wald test

The final test that we consider is based on the third of our difference measures, the difference between the MLE and the null parameter value. The test that comes from using this difference is called the **Wald test**, and takes its name from the statistician who first suggested it, Abraham Wald.

In Chapter 4 we discussed the properties of the MLE, and based on this discussion we know that if θ_0 is the true parameter value, that is the null hypothesis is true, then in large samples $\hat{\theta}$ is an observation from a distribution that is approximately normal, namely $N(\theta_0, I(\theta_0)^{-1})$. This approximate normality means that the observed statistic

$$t_W = \frac{D_3(\theta_0, \hat{\theta})^2}{I(\theta_0)^{-1}} = \frac{(\hat{\theta} - \theta_0)^2}{I(\theta_0)^{-1}}$$

is an observation from an approximate $\chi^2(1)$ distribution when the null hypothesis is true. As with t_{LR} and t_S, large values of the non-negative quantity t_W indicate that the sample is inconsistent with the null hypothesis. This again motivates a general hypothesis test applicable when n is large and there is just one parameter:

$$\textbf{Wald test}: \quad \text{reject } H_0 \quad \text{if} \quad t_W \geq \chi^2_{1-\alpha}(1).$$

As for the other two tests, this test will have significance level α.

Recall that in the extended example discussed in Chapter 5, we could either use the square of the standardised difference in proportions, and compare it to the χ^2 distribution, or use the standardised difference and compare it to the standard normal distribution. This was an example of a Wald test, and in general it is equivalent to using the standardised difference

$$s_W = \frac{\hat{\theta} - \theta_0}{\sqrt{I(\theta_0)^{-1}}}$$

together with the hypothesis test

$$\textbf{Wald test}: \quad \text{reject } H_0 \quad \text{if} \quad |s_W| \geq z_{1-\alpha/2}.$$

Written in this form, the Wald test has the most familiar form of the three tests, and arises in a number of basic hypothesis testing contexts, some of which will be discussed subsequently in this chapter. Writing the Wald test in this form also allows it to be adapted to one-sided hypothesis testing contexts. In particular, a simple null hypothesis and a one-sided alternative hypothesis

$$H_0 : \theta = \theta_0 \quad \text{versus} \quad H_1 : \theta > \theta_0$$

can be tested using

$$\textbf{Wald test (one-sided)}: \quad \text{reject } H_0 \quad \text{if} \quad s_W \geq z_{1-\alpha}.$$

A common modification of the Wald test is to use the estimated information $I(\hat{\theta})$, instead of the information under the null hypothesis $I(\theta_0)$, in the denominator of the test statistic. This means that the test statistics used to specify the Wald test become

$$t_{\mathrm{Wa}} = \frac{(\hat{\theta} - \theta_0)^2}{I(\hat{\theta})^{-1}} \quad \text{and} \quad s_{\mathrm{Wa}} = \frac{\hat{\theta} - \theta_0}{\sqrt{I(\hat{\theta})^{-1}}}.$$

When this modification is used we refer to the test as the **approximate Wald test**. It is often used because, while providing a reasonable approximation to the regular Wald test, it allows convenient calculation of the test statistics when the estimate $\hat{\theta}$ and its standard error $\sqrt{I(\hat{\theta})^{-1}}$ are available.

Example 6.3 Continuing from Examples 6.1 and 6.2 the Wald test statistic is

$$t_{\mathrm{W}} = \frac{(0.0494 - 0.5)^2}{I(0.05)^{-1}} = 0.079$$

which is very similar to the other tests, although not identical, and would not lead to rejection of the null hypothesis when compared with the critical value 3.84. Note that the approximate Wald test would involve using $I(0.0494)$ instead of $I(0.05)$ in the above calculation which yields a test statistic of $t_{\mathrm{Wa}} = 0.081$, identical to the score test statistic. Indeed, in this context it can be shown that the score test and the approximate Wald test are algebraically identical, although this is not always the case.

6.5 Comparison of the three approaches

As presented above, all three methods of constructing hypothesis tests are approximate methods applicable in large samples. While they were each derived from different perspectives, a series expansion of the log-likelihood function can be used to show that all three tests actually approximate each other. This generally means that in situations where the sample is large enough for one method to be applicable, the other methods will also usually be applicable and should give similar results. Nonetheless, there are some noteworthy practical and theoretical differences between the tests that we summarise in this section.

In some limited cases it is possible to determine the exact distributions of the test statistics, without relying on the large sample approximation. In this case the test statistics could be compared with the exact distributions, rather than the χ^2 approximations used above, and the associated hypothesis tests may perform better. In practice though, biostatistical analyses commonly make use of the tests as presented above. When the exact distributions of the test statistics are known, the likelihood ratio test has a theoretical advantage in that it is always the most powerful test when testing a simple null hypothesis versus a simple alternative hypothesis. This is an important result in theoretical statistics, known as the **Neyman-Pearson lemma**, but in practice this type of hypothesis test is rarely of interest. For the usual situation of testing a simple null hypothesis versus a composite alternative hypothesis, none of the three tests is always more powerful than the others. In some circumstances one method may be more powerful while in other circumstances another method may be more powerful. Since the three methods can be expected to approximate each other in large samples, if substantial differences in the P-values of the three methods arise, it is likely caused by the large sample approximation not being applicable. This may indicate the need to investigate exact methods of inference, and we will return to such methods on Chapter 8.

In practice, deciding which method to use in any given situation is largely a matter of convenience. When testing an hypothesis about a single parameter, the approximate Wald test using the estimated information is commonly the most convenient, especially when the estimate and standard error are available. Although we have not discussed it yet, all of the methods generalise to hypotheses involving multiple parameters. In this case the likelihood ratio test is often the most convenient. This is particularly true where interest may rest on whether a group of parameters can be dropped from the model, such as occurs in some types of regression modelling. The score test has the computational advantage that the MLE does not actually have to be computed to compute the test statistic. Thus, in situations where an estimate is not needed, then the score test will often be the most convenient, although in practice it is usual to require an estimate and a confidence interval.

In addition to the large sample requirement, there are some other important limitations that apply to all three methods. These limitations essentially parallel those that were noted in Chapter 4 in relation to the properties of MLEs. The first of these is when the MLE of the parameter falls on the boundary of the parameter space, such as a value of 0 or 1 for a proportion. In this case the tests described above are not valid, and special exact methods specific to the context would need to be considered. The second relates to multiple parameter models, in which the number of parameters increases as the sample size increases. As discussed in Chapter 4, in this case the MLE may not be consistent, and the test methods described here are generally not valid.

As a final issue, note that computation of the score and Wald test statistics require the expected information to be computed. In some applications the expected information may be difficult to compute whereas the observed information may be straightforward to compute. In such situations it is standard to use the observed information as an approximation to the expected information, and calculate the test statistics based on the observed information (such an approximation can also be used for the calculation of standard errors for MLEs). This is relevant to the issue of how our tests are affected if we carry out a transformation of our parameter, or a reparameterisation, which is a concept that we discussed in Chapter 4. When the expected information is used, the score test will lead to exactly the same result if we carry out a reparameterisation, whereas when the observed information is used the score test will change when we reparameterise. The Wald test will always change when we reparameterise, whether we use the observed or expected information, while the likelihood ratio test never changes when we reparameterise. Ideally we would like our test not to change if we measure our parameter on a different scale, so this represents an advantage of the likelihood ratio test over the other two tests. When taken together with the fact that the likelihood ratio test has the theoretical advantage of being the most powerful test for comparing simple hypotheses, the likelihood ratio test is often seen as being the more desirable of the three. However, this will not always necessarily be the case, and all three tests are generally valid and acceptable in the vast majority of situations encountered in practice.

6.6 Multiple parameters

In Chapters 3 and 4 we discussed likelihood functions and maximum likelihood estimation based on models with multiple parameters. When our model depends on a vector of p parameters, $\theta = (\theta_1, \ldots, \theta_p)$, all of the hypothesis testing methods described above can be generalised to accommodate this extra complexity. However, the details of the generalisation, and the convenience of implementing it, will depend on the nature of the hypotheses being tested. In particular, it will depend on whether or not we are interested in testing hypotheses about all of the p parameters. Sometimes one parameter from among the vector of p parameters may be our primary interest, while in other situations we may be interested in more than one parameter but not the entire collection of p parameters. This means that when we generalise our three testing approaches to allow for multiple parameters, we need to consider a range of different types of hypotheses that may be of interest.

With the above discussion in mind, we will be concerned with the following three common scenarios for testing hypotheses about a vector of parameters $\theta = (\theta_1, \ldots, \theta_p)$:

1. hypotheses about all of the p parameters;

2. hypotheses about just one of the p parameters;

3. hypotheses about some, but not all, of the p parameters.

The likelihood ratio, score and Wald testing methods discussed previously in this chapter can all be extended to allow for any of the three hypothesis types listed above. For testing hypotheses about all of the parameters simultaneously, the generalisations of each of the testing methods will be presented below. We will not consider all of the generalisations for the other two types of hypotheses, but will focus on the most convenient and useful of the testing methods in each case. The next three sections will consider each of the three types of hypotheses listed above.

6.7 Hypotheses about all parameters

Previously in this chapter we discussed methods for testing whether a single parameter θ is equal to a particular value θ_0. In the context of a vector of parameters, $\theta = (\theta_1, \ldots, \theta_p)$, a natural generalisation of this is to test whether the vector θ is equal to a particular value $\theta_0 = \left(\theta_0^{(1)}, \ldots, \theta_0^{(p)}\right)$. This amounts to testing an hypothesis about all of the parameters simultaneously. The statement of the null and alternative hypotheses in this situation looks similar to before, but now θ and θ_0 are p-dimensional vectors:

$$H_0 : \theta = \theta_0 \quad \text{versus} \quad H_1 : \theta \neq \theta_0.$$

When θ is a vector of p parameters, then all of the ingredients we used previously to define our test statistics become vector generalisations of their one parameter counterparts: the log-likelihood, $\ell(\theta)$, is a function of p variables; the MLE, $\hat{\theta} = (\hat{\theta}_1, \ldots, \hat{\theta}_p)$, and the score function, $S(\theta) = (S_1(\theta), \ldots, S_p(\theta))$, are p-dimensional vectors; and the information, $I(\theta)$, is a $p \times p$ matrix. While this can all be incorporated straightforwardly into a generalised form of each of our test statistics, an important change is that the generalised test statistics no longer have a $\chi^2(1)$ distribution when the null hypothesis is true, they have a $\chi^2(p)$ distribution. Thus, rather than comparing our generalised test statistics with the $\chi^2(1)$ distribution, we will use the $\chi^2(p)$ distribution instead.

Bearing all this in mind, the specific forms of the multiple parameter tests can be stated in terms of the three generalised test statistics:

$$
\begin{aligned}
t_{\mathrm{LR}} &= 2\left[\ell(\hat{\theta}) - \ell(\theta_0)\right] \\
t_{\mathrm{S}} &= S(\theta_0)I(\theta_0)^{-1}S(\theta_0)^{\mathrm{T}} \\
t_{\mathrm{W}} &= (\hat{\theta} - \theta_0)I(\theta_0)(\hat{\theta} - \theta_0)^{\mathrm{T}}.
\end{aligned}
$$

Then, in each case, an hypothesis test with significance level α can be carried out by rejecting the null hypothesis if the test statistic exceeds the critical value $c = \chi^2_{1-\alpha}(p)$.

Notice that the likelihood ratio test statistic looks the same as it did in the one parameter case, but remember that the log-likelihood is now a function of p variables rather than one. The form of the Wald and score test statistics is in each case a matrix generalisation of the form of these test statistics in the one parameter case. Calculation of these test statistics involves matrix transpose, multiplication and inversion. As was the case in the one parameter test, the information used in the definition of the Wald test will often be approximated by the estimated information $I(\hat{\theta})$, to produce a more convenient approximate version of the Wald test.

6.8 Hypotheses about one parameter

Often in multiple parameter situations there is one parameter that is of primary concern, while the other parameters are of only secondary concern. It may then be of interest to test an hypothesis about the parameter of primary concern, without saying anything about the other parameters. That is, if θ_j is our primary concern from among the p parameters $(\theta_1, \ldots, \theta_p)$, and $\theta_0^{(j)}$ is the null value for θ_j, then our null and alternative hypotheses can be stated as:

$$H_0 : \theta_j = \theta_0^{(j)} \quad \text{versus} \quad H_1 : \theta_j \neq \theta_0^{(j)}.$$

In situations where our primary interest rests with one parameter θ_j, we will usually have available the parameter estimate, $\hat{\theta}_j$, and its estimated standard error, $\text{se}(\hat{\theta}_j)$. When this is the case, an approximate Wald test is the most convenient way to conduct an hypothesis test concerning this single parameter. In this case the test statistic is

$$t_{\text{Wa}} = \frac{(\hat{\theta}_j - \theta_0^{(j)})^2}{\text{se}(\hat{\theta}_j)^2}$$

which is compared with the $\chi^2(1)$ distribution, and the null hypothesis is rejected if t_{W} exceeds the critical value $c = \chi^2_{1-\alpha}(1)$.

Notice that by using the estimated standard error in the denominator of t_{Wa}, the above approach makes use of the estimated information rather than the information under the null hypothesis. That is why this test is referred to as an approximate Wald test, because it is analogous to the approximate Wald test discussed in Section 6.4. The test statistic could alternatively be computed using the information under the null hypothesis, making the test analogous to the regular Wald test, but this will usually be less convenient and is therefore not the way such tests are generally carried out. One notable exception to this is the situation discussed in detail in the extended example of Chapter 5, the comparison of two proportions.

Analogously to the discussion for the one parameter case, the square root of t_{Wa} can equivalently be compared with the standard normal distribution. This approach is useful when carrying out a one-sided test, as was explained in Section 6.4.

The approximate Wald test described above is probably the most common way of conducting a test concerning a single parameter of primary concern from among a larger number of parameters. Nonetheless, such tests are also sometimes conducted using the other testing methods, particularly the likelihood ratio test. We will not write down the explicit form of these tests here, but for the likelihood ratio test the approach for a single parameter is just a special case of the approach that we will discuss in the next section for a subgroup of parameters. This will be illustrated in the next section.

Example 6.4 Consider the stroke incidence study without the assumption that the two diet groups have the same event rate, and suppose we are interested in testing whether there is a difference in stroke rates between the two groups. Based on the data used in the extended example of Chapter 4, the 484 stroke events were split 245 and 239 into the low and high salt intake groups, respectively. Likewise, the 9805 person-years of total follow-up were split 5980 and 3825 into the two diet groups. Letting the stroke rate in the low intake group be λ_1 and in the high intake group be $\gamma\lambda_1$, then we have a two-parameter model in terms of λ_1 and γ. Our primary interest is the rate ratio parameter γ, and we wish to test

$$H_0 : \gamma = 1 \quad \text{versus} \quad H_1 : \gamma \neq 1$$

without saying anything about λ_1. In Chapter 4 we derived the MLEs $\hat{\lambda}_1 = 0.0410$ and $\hat{\gamma} = 1.52$, as well as a standard error estimate $\text{se}(\hat{\gamma}) = 0.138$. It follows that the approximate Wald test statistic is

$$t_{\text{Wa}} = \frac{(1.52 - 1)^2}{0.138^2} = 14.20$$

which is greater than the critical value $\chi^2(1) = 3.84$ and would lead us to reject the null hypothesis at the 5% significance level, with $P = 0.0002$. That is, we would conclude that there is evidence that the stroke rates in the two dietary groups are different.

6.9   Hypotheses about some parameters

It is often the case that we are interested in testing hypotheses involving some sub-group of the p parameters. As discussed later, this arises most commonly in statistical model building where we may be interested in whether a collection of parameters can all be dropped from the model. The context of testing hypotheses about a subgroup of parameters leads to a very general approach to hypothesis testing. In particular, it provides a generalisation of the situations discussed in the previous two sections: if the subgroup of parameters includes just one parameter then we are in the situation discussed in Section 6.8; whereas, if the subgroup of parameters includes all of the p parameters then we are in the situation discussed in Section 6.7. However, importantly, it also covers situations intermediate to these two extremes.

The most common way to test hypotheses about a subgroup of parameters is using a generalised version of the likelihood ratio test. Suppose the parameter vector θ can be divided into two groups of parameters $\theta = \left(\theta^{[1]}, \theta^{[2]}\right)$, where $\theta^{[1]}$ is a vector of $p - q$ parameters and $\theta^{[2]}$ is a vector of q parameters. For example, we might have $\theta^{[1]} = (\theta_1, \theta_2)$ and $\theta^{[2]} = (\theta_3, \ldots, \theta_p)$. If we are interested in testing hypotheses about the parameters contained in $\theta^{[1]}$ without saying anything about the parameters contained in $\theta^{[2]}$, then for a vector of $p - q$ values $\theta_0^{[1]}$, the hypotheses are:

$$H_0 : \theta^{[1]} = \theta_0^{[1]} \quad \text{versus} \quad H_1 : \theta^{[1]} \neq \theta_0^{[1]}.$$

We use the term **full model** to refer to the model involving all p parameters. We use the term **null model** to refer to the model involving the q parameters contained in $\theta^{[2]}$, with the other parameters assumed to follow the null hypothesis $\theta^{[1]} = \theta_0^{[1]}$. The full model has a log-likelihood function that is a function of all p parameters

$$\ell(\theta) = \ell\left(\left(\theta^{[1]}, \theta^{[2]}\right)\right).$$

The null model, which assumes the null hypothesis is true, has a log-likelihood function $\ell_0(\theta^{[2]})$ that is a function of the q parameters that do not occur in the null hypothesis. This is obtained by substituting the null hypothesis values for $\theta^{[1]}$ into the full log-likelihood, namely

$$\ell_0(\theta^{[2]}) = \ell\left(\left(\theta_0^{[1]}, \theta^{[2]}\right)\right).$$

The maximum value achieved by the null log-likelihood ℓ_0 will be no greater than that achieved by the full log-likelihood ℓ. Furthermore, the magnitude of the difference between the two is a measure of the extent to which the full model provides a better explanation of the sample than the null model. That is, it provides a measure of the extent to which the sample departs from the null hypothesis.

To describe a test based on the above log-likelihood difference, let $\hat{\theta}^{[2]}$ be the value of $\theta^{[2]}$ that maximises ℓ_0, in other words the MLE of $\theta^{[2]}$ under the null hypothesis. That is, $\ell_0(\hat{\theta}^{[2]})$ is the maximum value achieved by the log-likelihood corresponding to the null model. Furthermore, let $\hat{\theta}$ be the MLE from the full model, so that $\ell(\hat{\theta})$ is the maximum value achieved by the log-likelihood corresponding to the full model. Then the likelihood ratio test statistic becomes

$$t_{\text{LR}} = 2\left[\ell(\hat{\theta}) - \ell_0(\hat{\theta}^{[2]})\right]$$

and the likelihood ratio test is

Likelihood ratio test : reject H_0 if $t_{\text{LR}} \geq \chi^2_{1-\alpha}(p-q)$.

Notice that the χ^2 distribution used in this likelihood ratio test has $p - q$ degrees of freedom, being the number of parameters that are involved in the null hypothesis. In the special case that $\theta^{[1]}$ consists of just one parameter, then the above likelihood ratio test is analogous (but not identical) to the one parameter Wald test described in the previous section. In the special case that $\theta^{[1]}$ consists of all p parameters, $\theta^{[1]} = \theta$, then the above test corresponds to the likelihood ratio test involving all parameters as described in Section 6.7.

The most common situation in which this type of test is used is for testing whether a model can be simplified by removing a subgroup of parameters from the model. This often occurs in regression modelling, where the goal may be to assess whether a collection of predictors can be removed from the model by having their coefficients all set to zero. It also occurs in tests of interaction, in which the goal is to test whether all parameters involved in a multi-way interaction can be removed from the model.

Another application of this type of test is in situations where we have nuisance parameters. Thus, $\theta^{[1]}$ may be interpreted as the collection of parameters of interest, while $\theta^{[2]}$ is interpreted as the collection of nuisance parameters. In this case the likelihood ratio test described above is equivalent to conducting a likelihood ratio test based on the profile log-likelihood, which was discussed in Chapter 3. Finally, it should be noted that the methods discussed in the section can be extended even further to provide a likelihood ratio test for testing a general composite null hypothesis against a general composite alternative hypothesis. This makes the likelihood ratio test a very powerful approach in multiple parameter settings. A detailed illustration of the methods discussed in this section is provided in Section 6.11.5 of the extended example.

6.10   Test-based confidence intervals

In Chapter 5 we stressed the importance of accompanying an hypothesis test with a confidence interval for the parameter under study, and described the correspondence between confidence intervals and hypothesis tests. We now look at how the test methods described in this chapter can be used to provide confidence intervals. The basic idea is that hypothesis tests reject the null hypothesis when the parameter estimate is "far" from the value specified by the null hypothesis. Thus, for any of the three hypothesis test methods, the range of parameter values that would not be rejected corresponds to the range of plausible values for the parameter, or in other words, a confidence interval.

To describe this correspondence, consider a one-dimensional parameter θ. If the model actually involves more than one parameter, then for the purpose of this discussion θ can be interpreted as one component of the vector of parameters for which a confidence interval is desired. For testing the null hypothesis $H_0 : \theta = \theta_0$, each of the three test statistics is a function of the value θ_0, for example $t_{LR} = t_{LR}(\theta_0)$. The range of values of θ_0 for which the null hypothesis would not be rejected can be interpreted as a $100(1 - \alpha)\%$ confidence interval. This range of values corresponds to the set

$$\{\theta_0 : t_{LR}(\theta_0) < \chi^2_{1-\alpha}(1)\}.$$

This definition can also be used based on the test statistics $t_S(\theta_0)$ and $t_W(\theta_0)$ to obtain alternative definitions of a confidence interval for θ.

The question now arises, how do these test-based confidence intervals relate to the usual confidence interval:

$$\hat{\theta} \pm z_{1-\alpha/2} \times \text{se}\left(\hat{\theta}\right).$$

In fact, it can be shown that the usual confidence interval corresponds to using a Wald test statistic in the test-based definition. In particular, the approximate version of the Wald statistic is used, based on the estimated information rather than the information under the null hypothesis. The definitions obtained using the other test statistics will lead to different confidence intervals, and may have more accurate coverage probabilities. In general, however, they will approximate the usual method of confidence interval estimation and will be somewhat less convenient to calculate.

Importantly, the same test-based definition of a confidence interval can be used even if the parameter is a vector rather than a single parameter. In this case, however, the resulting confidence "interval" is actually a multi-dimensional region referred to as a **confidence region**. Such a confidence region represents a region within which we are confident that all parameters lie simultaneously, and has a similar repeated sampling interpretation as a confidence interval for a single parameter. The construction of a confidence region for more than one parameter will be illustrated in the extended example.

Example 6.5 In this example we will consider a test-based confidence interval for the one-parameter stroke incidence example discussed in Example 6.1. In the extended example to follow we will study a more detailed example in which a confidence region for multiple parameters is considered. Based on the one-parameter log-likelihood function from Example 6.1, the test-based 95% confidence interval using the likelihood ratio test is the interval

$$
\begin{aligned}
\left\{\lambda_0 : t_{LR}(\lambda_0) < 3.84\right\} &= \left\{\lambda_0 : \ell(\lambda_0) > \ell(\hat{\lambda}) - 3.84 \times 0.5\right\} \\
&= \left\{\lambda_0 : 484\log(\lambda_0) - 9805\lambda_0 > -1942.064\right\}.
\end{aligned}
$$

By plotting out the log-likelihood function $\ell(\lambda)$ and marking a line at the value -1942.064, it can be seen how the test-based confidence interval is related to the log-likelihood function. This correspondence is presented in Figure 6.1, where it can be seen that the confidence interval corresponds to all parameter values that lead to a sufficiently high log-likelihood. That is, the confidence interval consists of all parameter values that have sufficiently high support from the sample. Equivalently, we could have plotted the test statistic $t_{LR}(\lambda_0)$ as a function of λ_0 and identified the range that leads to values less than 3.84 (see Exercise 2). Based on Figure 6.1, the test-based 95% confidence interval is $(0.045, 0.054)$. This is identical to the 95% confidence interval calculated in Chapter 4 using the usual method, although in general the two are not numerically equivalent.

6.11 Extended example

In this example we consider a study in which the outcome is the time from disease progression until death for individuals with end stage terminal cancer. The main objective is to illustrate the derivation and use of the different testing methods described in this chapter. We will begin by considering a single study group and use

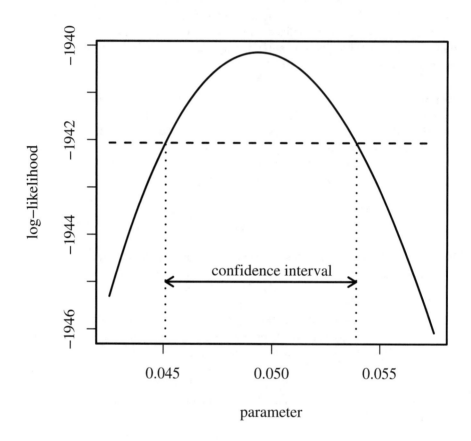

FIGURE 6.1
Test-based 95% confidence interval using the likelihood ratio test in the stroke incidence example

a one-parameter model based on the exponential distribution. Using this model we will derive each of the different types of test statistics discussed in this chapter, for testing a null hypothesis that the mortality rate is equal to a particular number determined from historical data. We will then generalise the context to a randomised study comparing three treatment groups: no treatment; radiotherapy alone; or the combination of radiotherapy and chemotherapy. Using a three parameter model we will consider tests of various hypotheses concerning the equality of mortality rates in different treatment groups. There are some important assumptions in this illustrative example that are worth keeping in mind. Firstly, as in previous contexts, we assume that the parametric model based on the exponential distribution is appropriate, but in practice this would need to be assessed. In addition, it will be assumed that all participants die prior to the end of the study. This assumption is reasonable in the present context of end stage cancer; however, in many other settings involving the study of the time to death the study may end before all participants die. This leads to the need for so-called "censored" data methods, also called survival analysis, which allow for the incomplete observation of some individuals in the study. Survival analysis is an important topic in biostatistics which is beyond our scope, but an introduction is provided in some of the general methods texts discussed in Appendix 3, such as Armitage et al. (2002).

6.11.1 Survival with end stage cancer

Consider a randomised trial of the treatment of patients with terminal cancer. Three potential approaches to caring for such patients are studied, involving three groups of n patients with end stage cancer, leading to $3n$ patients in total. The groups are labelled 1–3, and consist of patients who were randomised to receive one of three treatments: (1) no treatment other than regular palliative care; (2) radiotherapy alone; or (3) the combination of radiotherapy and chemotherapy. The outcome is the time from progression into end stage cancer until the patients dies, and is denoted $x_1, \ldots, x_n$ for the no treatment group, $y_1, \ldots, y_n$ for the radiotherapy alone group, and $z_1, \ldots, z_n$ for the combination therapy group. The survival time for each patient is modelled using an exponential distribution, as described in Appendix 1. In particular, we assume that the survival times for each group have the following distributions:

$$\text{Group 1} : \exp(\lambda) \quad \text{Group 2} : \exp(\gamma_2 \lambda) \quad \text{Group 3} : \exp(\gamma_3 \lambda).$$

Thus, overall we have a three-parameter model involving the vector of parameters $\theta = (\lambda, \gamma_2, \gamma_3)$. The parameter λ is interpreted as a "baseline" mortality rate under no treatment, while γ_j is the mortality rate ratio of the active treatment group j, compared to the no treatment group. Values less than 1 for γ_2 or γ_3 indicate a reduced mortality rate, while values in excess of 1 indicate an increased mortality rate, relative to the no treatment group.

Based on historical data it is believed that these patients would live for an average of 4 months in the absence of treatment, or in other words, the mortality rate is 3.0 per person per year. One problem that we will consider is whether there is evidence of a difference between the mortality rate in our control group and the historical mor-

TABLE 6.1

Mean survival time (months) after progression into end stage cancer

	No treatment	Radiotherapy	Combination
Sample size	100	100	100
Mean survival	4.8	7.4	5.6

tality rate. In practice this is likely to be a secondary consideration in a randomised trial, since there are many reasons why there might be inconsistencies with historical data. It does, however, provide a useful illustration of the various types of tests in a simplified context. Of more interest are hypotheses concerning whether the active treatment groups have different survival patterns to the control group receiving no treatment. We will consider this in two ways: separate tests of whether the active treatment groups differ from the control group, and a test of whether there is an overall difference between the treatment groups. Thus, there are three types of tests that we will consider:

1. Based on the control group only, test whether the mortality rate is different to the historical rate of 3.0 per person per year;

2. Based on data from all three groups, test whether radiotherapy alone results in a different mortality rate to no treatment, and whether the combination of chemotherapy and radiotherapy results in a different mortality rate to no treatment. This involves two separate tests, and allows an assessment of whether either of the active treatment arms extends life relative to no treatment;

3. Based on data from all three groups, test whether there is any difference in the mortality rates among the three treatment groups. This involves one test, and is often the primary hypothesis test in a randomised trial involving more than two treatment groups. The tests described under item 2 above would usually be carried out after this "global" test of difference.

We will consider the above testing problems based on the observed data described in Table 6.1.

6.11.2   Comparison with an historical rate

In order to compare the mortality rate of the control group with the historical mortality rate, we consider each of the following four tests: (i) likelihood ratio test; (ii) score test; (iii) Wald test; and (iv) approximate Wald test. Recall that the approximate Wald test evaluates the information at the MLE of the parameter, rather than the null hypothesis value of the parameter. In each case, the hypotheses under consideration are as follows, reflecting a desire to test whether an historical mortality rate of $\lambda_0 = 3.0$ per person per year is consistent with the observed sample:

$$H_0 : \lambda = 3.0 \quad \text{versus} \quad H_1 : \lambda \neq 3.0.$$

Using data from the control group only, the survival time of individual i, x_i, is an observation from an exponential distribution with probability density function $f(x_i; \lambda) = \lambda \exp(-\lambda x_i)$. It follows that the log-likelihood function associated with the sample $x_1, \ldots, x_{100}$ is

$$\ell(\lambda) = 100 \log(\lambda) - \lambda \sum_{i=1}^{100} x_i,$$

which leads to the score function

$$S(\lambda) = \frac{d\ell(\lambda)}{d\lambda} = \frac{100}{\lambda} - \sum_{i=1}^{100} x_i.$$

Solving the score equation $S(\lambda) = 0$ leads to the MLE

$$\hat{\lambda} = \frac{100}{\sum_{i=1}^{100} x_i} = \frac{1}{\bar{x}}$$

and taking the derivative of the score function leads to the information (both expected and observed)

$$I(\lambda) = \frac{100}{\lambda^2}.$$

The four equations above supply all the quantities that we need to specify each of the desired tests. In particular, the following numerical calculations are required to construct the four test statistics, using the fact that $\bar{x} = 0.4$ years:

$$\lambda_0 = 3.0 \qquad \ell(\lambda_0) = -10.14 \qquad S(\lambda_0) = -6.67 \qquad I(\lambda_0) = 11.11$$

$$\hat{\lambda} = 2.5 \qquad \ell(\hat{\lambda}) = -8.37 \qquad S(\hat{\lambda}) = 0 \qquad I(\hat{\lambda}) = 16.0.$$

These calculations lead to the following values for the four test statistics:

$$\text{Likelihood ratio} \quad : \quad t_{LR} = 2\left[\ell(\hat{\lambda}) - \ell(\lambda_0)\right] = \mathbf{3.54}$$

$$\text{Score} \quad : \quad t_S = \frac{S(\lambda_0)^2}{I(\lambda_0)} = \mathbf{4.00}$$

$$\text{Wald} \quad : \quad t_W = (\hat{\lambda} - \lambda_0)^2 I(\lambda_0) = \mathbf{2.78}$$

$$\text{Wald (approximate)} \quad : \quad t_{Wa} = (\hat{\lambda} - \lambda_0)^2 I(\hat{\lambda}) = \mathbf{4.00}.$$

Notice that the score test statistic and the approximate Wald test statistic have the same value. In fact, it can be shown that for this particular model these test statistics are algebraically identical, although this is not always the case. In view of this equivalence for the present context, we will consider only the likelihood ratio, score and Wald tests below. In each case the test statistics are compared with a $\chi^2(1)$ distribution. Using a significance level of 5%, the critical value for each test statistic is $\chi^2_{0.95}(1) = 3.84$, and the P-value associated with each test is obtained by calculating the probability that a $\chi^2(1)$ random variable exceeds the observed value of the test statistic, e.g. $P = \Pr(\chi^2(1) \geq 3.54)$ for the likelihood ratio test. By comparing the observed test statistics with the critical value it can be seen that the score test would reject the null hypothesis but the other two tests would not reject the null hypothesis. The associated P-values for each test are:

$$\text{Likelihood ratio} \quad : \quad P = \mathbf{0.060}$$
$$\text{Score} \quad : \quad P = \mathbf{0.046}$$
$$\text{Wald} \quad : \quad P = \mathbf{0.095}.$$

Before attempting to explore the reason why the three tests yield different qualitative conclusions, it is important to emphasise that the quantitative difference between the three P-values is not great, and whichever test is used the result is on the border of significance and non-significance. In particular, it is important not to read too much into the fact that one test may lead to the rejection of the null hypothesis with a P-value of 0.046, while another test may lead to non-rejection of the null hypothesis with a P-value of 0.060. In reality these two P-values are indistinguishable, and their different qualitative conclusion arises only because of the arbitrary choice of 5% as the cut-off for statistical significance. Rather than relying solely on whether the cut-off of 5% has been achieved, a better approach is to emphasise the magnitude of the P-value, which in this case leads to the suggestion that the mortality rate may be lower in this population than the historical rate, however, a strong conclusion is not possible.

Recall that the hypothesis tested above would not be the most important hypothesis in this study, as the comparison of mortality rates between groups would be primary. Furthermore, even if we did conclude that there is a significant departure from the historical mortality rate, the reason for this is not clear — it could be improvements in the background standard of care, differences between the historical patients and those included in this study, or many other explanations. However, the present example does provide a useful illustration of the application of the tests, which will be continued in the next section, and then followed by an assessment of the comparative hypotheses in later sections.

6.11.3   Repeated sampling properties

It is often a good idea to pre-specify the type of test that will be used, so that it cannot be claimed that the method has been chosen opportunistically after the results were known. In this case, it is useful to be able to assess the properties of the tests, so that the "best" method can be chosen as the one that will be used. Previously in this chapter we noted that none of the three approaches will be the best in all situations. We now consider a more extensive comparison of the three tests to help explain the manner in which they differ for this particular setting. To do this we consider the repeated sampling interpretation of the three tests, and in particular their tendency to reject the null hypothesis in a large number of identical studies repeated in the same way as that described above. By considering a range of assumptions about the true underlying mortality rate, this amounts to considering a simulation-based assessment of the power and significance level of the three tests.

Consider a large number of identical hypothetical studies (in this case 10,000) carried out on the same population of end stage cancer patients, in which the survival time after progressing into end stage cancer is observed in a sample of 100 patients. Assuming that the mortality rate in this population of cancer patients is 3.0 per person per year (i.e. that the null hypothesis is true), Figure 6.2 displays the observed values of the likelihood ratio test statistic for the 10,000 studies. Also shown are the frequencies that would be expected assuming the likelihood ratio statistic has a $\chi^2(1)$ distribution. Analogous graphs for the score and Wald tests look very similar to Figure 6.2. In light of Figure 6.2, it can be seen that the distributions of the test statistics closely approximate a $\chi^2(1)$ distribution, so that the large sample approximation seems reasonable. The proportion of studies where the test statistic exceeds the critical value of $\chi_{0.95}(1) = 3.84$ corresponds to the proportion of type I errors, or false positives. This is close to 0.05 for all three tests, which is what it should be given that the critical value has been determined so as to yield a significance level of 0.05. The actual values are 0.047 for the likelihood ratio and score tests, and 0.053 for the Wald test.

Since all three tests behave appropriately in terms of controlling the chance that the null hypothesis will be rejected when in fact it is true, it is of interest to compare how the three tests behave when the null hypothesis is not true. Consider a range of different hypothetical end stage cancer populations in which the mortality rate ranges from 1.0 to 5.0 per person per year. Suppose 10,000 studies were conducted on each of these populations, and the three tests were used to test the null hypothesis that the mortality rate is 3.0. Then, for a particular population (that is, a particular assumption about the mortality rate) the proportion of Wald tests that reject the null hypothesis indicates the power of the Wald test, and likewise for the other testing methods. Figure 6.3 plots this proportion as a function of the assumed mortality rate, for each of the three tests. This plot is sometimes referred to as the **empirical power function**, since it is a simulation-based approximation to the power function.

Figure 6.3 shows that no single test provides the greatest power for all possible values of the underlying mortality rate. For a population in which the true mortality rate is lower than the null hypothesis value of 3.0, the score test is the most powerful of the three tests, in that it will reject the null hypothesis in a greater proportion of studies sampled from this population. For a population in which the mortality rate is greater than the null hypothesis value of 3.0, the Wald test is the most powerful of the three tests. The likelihood ratio test is not the most powerful for any value of the mortality rate, but when considered across the whole range of possible values for the population mortality rate it might be considered to provide the most robust power function, in that it is the second most powerful test for all mortality rates. Notice that all three tests have a power of approximately 0.05 when the population mortality rate is equal to the null hypothesis value of 3.0, which is equivalent to our earlier observation that all three tests have a significance level of approximately 0.05.

The above power comparisons are consistent with our earlier analysis results in that the data led to an estimated mortality rate that was lower than the null hypothesis value of 3.0, and the score test provided the most significant *P*-value, followed by the likelihood ratio test and then the Wald test. In a two-sided hypothesis situation, where

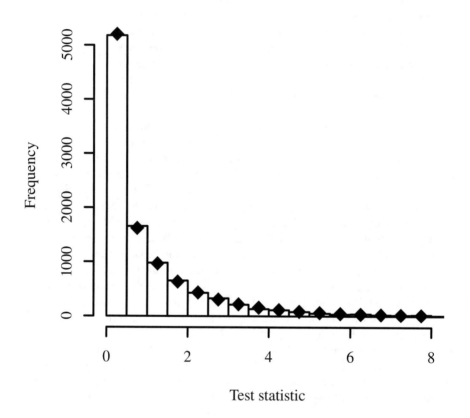

FIGURE 6.2
Histogram of the likelihood ratio test statistic in 10,000 studies with the expected $\chi^2(1)$ frequencies shown by diamonds (score and Wald test results look similar)

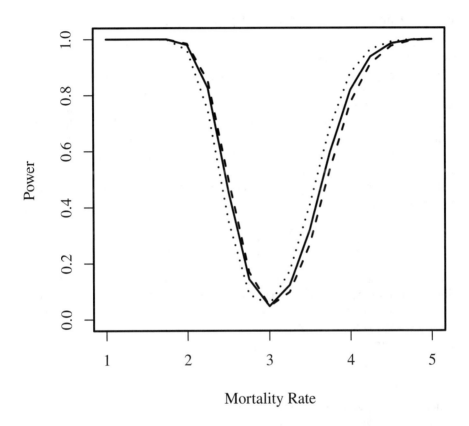

FIGURE 6.3
Proportion of studies rejecting the null hypothesis (power) in 10,000 simulations of studies on populations with various mortality rates (per person per year). Simulations were conducted for 17 mortality rates in the range 1.0–5.0, and the power functions were plotted by joining the points for each of the likelihood ratio (solid line), score (dashed line) and Wald (dotted line) tests

mortality rates above and below the null hypothesis value of 3.0 are both plausible, the likelihood ratio test would seem to have the best overall power function. However, if mortality rates below 3.0 were anticipated then a score test might be preferred. In either case the results of our analysis based on these two tests are highly consistent, and the fact that they led to *P*-values on either side of 0.05 should not be over-interpreted.

6.11.4   Comparison with a control rate

We now consider tests of whether the active treatment groups, radiotherapy alone or radiotherapy plus chemotherapy, have mortality rates that differ from the control group receiving no treatment. Since both of these treatments have potential toxicities as well as potential beneficial effects, two-sided tests are appropriate, allowing for the possibility of both decreases or increases in mortality. In this section we consider separate comparisons of the active treatment mortality rates with the control mortality rate, as described in the second of our testing problems at the beginning of this extended example. Thus, recalling that γ_2 and γ_3 are the mortality rate ratios for comparing the no treatment group with the radiotherapy and radiotherapy plus chemotherapy groups, respectively, we are interested in separate tests of the following two sets of hypotheses:

(1)	$H_0 : \gamma_2 = 1$	versus	$H_1 : \gamma_2 \neq 1$
(2)	$H_0 : \gamma_3 = 1$	versus	$H_1 : \gamma_3 \neq 1$.

There are a number of ways in which this can be done, however, as described in Section 6.8 the most common way is based on an approximate Wald test using the estimated standard errors associated with the parameter estimates. Using this approach, the test statistics for the two tests are:

$$\textbf{(1)} \quad t_{\text{Wa}} = \frac{\left(\hat{\gamma}_2 - 1\right)^2}{\text{se}\left(\hat{\gamma}_2\right)^2} \qquad \textbf{(2)} \quad t_{\text{Wa}} = \frac{\left(\hat{\gamma}_3 - 1\right)^2}{\text{se}\left(\hat{\gamma}_3\right)^2}$$

which in each case must be compared with the critical value $\chi^2_{0.95}(1) = 3.84$ to achieve significance levels of 0.05.

Based on the data from all three treatment groups, together with the exponential distributions described earlier in this section, the full log-likelihood function is:

$$\ell(\theta) = \ell(\lambda, \gamma_2, \gamma_3) \quad = \quad 300 \log(\lambda) + 100 \log(\gamma_2) + 100 \log(\gamma_3)$$
$$-\lambda \left(\sum_{i=1}^{100} x_i + \gamma_2 \sum_{i=1}^{100} y_i + \gamma_3 \sum_{i=1}^{100} z_i \right).$$

Differentiating this log-likelihood with respect to each of the three parameters leads to the following MLEs for the data described in Table 6.1:

$$\hat{\lambda} = \frac{1}{\bar{x}} = 2.5 \qquad \hat{\gamma}_2 = \frac{\bar{x}}{\bar{y}} = 0.65 \qquad \hat{\gamma}_2 = \frac{\bar{x}}{\bar{z}} = 0.86.$$

Similarly, differentiating the log-likelihood twice with respect to each parameter leads to the expected information matrix $I(\theta)$ and its value $I(\hat{\theta})$ when evaluated at the MLE:

$$I(\theta) = 100 \times \begin{bmatrix} \frac{3}{\lambda^2} & \frac{1}{\gamma_2\lambda} & \frac{1}{\gamma_3\lambda} \\ \frac{1}{\gamma_2\lambda} & \frac{1}{\gamma_2^2} & 0 \\ \frac{1}{\gamma_3\lambda} & 0 & \frac{2}{\gamma_3^2} \end{bmatrix} \quad I(\hat{\theta}) = \begin{bmatrix} 48.00 & 61.54 & 46.51 \\ 61.54 & 236.69 & 0 \\ 46.51 & 0 & 135.21 \end{bmatrix}.$$

Taking the inverse of $I(\hat{\theta})$ leads to the standard error estimates $\mathrm{se}(\hat{\gamma}_2) = \sqrt{0.00845}$ and $\mathrm{se}(\hat{\gamma}_3) = \sqrt{0.0148}$, which yield the following Wald test statistics based on the previous formulae:

$$\textbf{(1)} \quad t_{\mathrm{Wa}} = \frac{(0.65-1)^2}{0.00845} = 14.50 \qquad \textbf{(2)} \quad t_{\mathrm{Wa}} = \frac{(0.86-1)^2}{0.0148} = 1.32.$$

The first test statistic exceeds the critical value of 3.84, with $P = 0.0001$, while the second test statistic is less than the critical value with $P = 0.25$. It is therefore reasonable to conclude based on these data that radiotherapy alone extends the life of end stage cancer patients. There is insufficient evidence in these data to conclude that the combination of radiotherapy and chemotherapy extends the life of such patients. Note that while some of the computational details of the above calculations have been omitted, they follow the same pattern as the methods described in Chapter 4 for deriving MLEs and their standard errors.

Since we have conducted two tests, each with a type I error probability (significance level) of $\alpha = 0.05$, the probability that at least one of the tests is significant purely by chance will be greater than 0.05. This phenomenon was studied in the exercises in Chapter 5. In particular, we referred to a correction for this multiple testing problem, called the Bonferroni correction, which in our case would require that we conduct each or our two tests using a significance level of $\alpha/2 = 0.025$. This would ensure that the probability of at least one test being significant purely by chance does not exceed $\alpha = 0.05$. Even with this correction, however, we see that the comparison involving the radiotherapy group would remain statistically significant, since the P-value is less than 0.025. In general, when more than one test is carried out then a correction for multiple testing, such as the Bonferroni correction, should be considered.

6.11.5 Global test of mortality difference

Although the separate comparisons described above will often be of most interest, in practice it is common in randomised studies having more than two treatment groups to carry out an initial "global" test of the hypothesis of equal mortality rates in all treatment groups. This allows a test for an overall difference in mortality rates without the multiple testing concerns described above. If the global test is not significant then the separate tests do not need to be carried out. This corresponds to the third of our testing problems described at the beginning of this extended example. It involves testing a null hypothesis about some but not all of the parameters in the model. The null and alternative hypotheses for a global test of treatment effect are:

$$\text{H}_0 : \gamma_2 = 1 \text{ and } \gamma_3 = 1 \quad \text{versus} \quad \text{H}_1 : \gamma_2 \neq 1 \text{ or } \gamma_3 \neq 1.$$

As described in this chapter, the usual way to carry out such an hypothesis test is using the likelihood ratio test. Using the notation that was introduced earlier, these hypotheses involve splitting the vector of parameters into two parts $\theta = (\theta^{[1]}, \theta^{[2]})$, where $\theta^{[1]} = (\gamma_2, \gamma_3)$ is the part that is involved in the hypotheses, and $\theta^{[2]} = \lambda$ is the part that the hypotheses do not concern. Thus, for $\theta_0^{[1]} = (1, 1)$, the hypotheses may be rewritten as

$$\text{H}_0 : \theta^{[1]} = \theta_0^{[1]} \quad \text{versus} \quad \text{H}_1 : \theta^{[1]} \neq \theta_0^{[1]}.$$

The log-likelihood associated with the full model involving all three parameters was written down in the previous section, along with the MLEs under the full model. The log-likelihood associated with the null model, that is assuming the null hypothesis is true, corresponds to 300 observations from an exponential distribution with mortality rate λ:

$$\ell_0(\theta^{[2]}) = \ell_0(\lambda) = 300\log(\lambda) - \lambda\left(\sum_{i=1}^{100} x_i + \sum_{i=1}^{100} y_i + \sum_{i=1}^{100} z_i\right).$$

Thus, the MLE under the null model is

$$\hat{\theta}^{[2]} = \hat{\lambda} = \frac{3}{\bar{x} + \bar{y} + \bar{z}} = 2.02$$

which gives $\ell_0(\hat{\theta}^{[2]}) = -88.70$. This is the maximum value of the log-likelihood under the assumption that the null hypothesis is true. In contrast, the maximum value of the log-likelihood under the full model is $\ell(\hat{\theta}) = -83.82$, using the MLEs and the full log-likelihood described in the previous section.

The fact that $\ell(\hat{\theta}) > \ell_0(\hat{\theta}^{[2]})$ reflects the fact that the most supported parameter combination under the null hypothesis, $(\lambda, \gamma_2, \gamma_3) = (2.02, 1, 1)$, is less supported than the most supported parameter combination under the full model, $(\lambda, \gamma_2, \gamma_3) = (2.5, 0.65, 0.86)$. Indeed, it will always be the case that the MLEs under the full model have more support than the MLEs under the null model. The role of the likelihood ratio test is to assess whether this increase in the level of support is statistically significant, that is, to assess whether the data provide sufficient evidence to reject the null hypothesis. In this case the likelihood ratio test statistic is

$$t_{\text{LR}} = 2\left[\ell(\hat{\theta}) - \ell_0(\hat{\theta}^{[2]})\right] = 9.76$$

which must be compared with a critical value of $\chi^2_{0.95}(p - q) = \chi^2_{0.95}(2) = 5.99$, where $p = 3$ and $q = 1$ are the number of parameters under the full and null models, respectively. Thus, the null hypothesis would be rejected with $P = \text{Pr}(\chi^2_{0.95}(2) \geq 9.76) = 0.008$, and there is sufficient evidence to conclude that the mortality rates in the three treatment groups are not identical.

Since the above global test of equality of the mortality rates is statistically significant, it should be followed up with individual tests investigating how the rates differ. One common approach to this was described in the previous section, based on the Wald test. The likelihood ratio method employed above could also be used to provide separate tests of the null hypotheses $H_0 : \gamma_2 = 1$ and $H_0 : \gamma_3 = 1$, which would allow separate assessments of whether the active treatment rates differ from the control rate. It could also be used to test the null hypothesis $H_0 : \gamma_2 = \gamma_3$, which would allow an assessment of whether the two active treatment arms have different mortality rates. We will not discuss the details here, but we would expect them to be in relative agreement with the conclusions from the analogous Wald tests described previously, and the exercises will verify this.

6.11.6 Confidence intervals

We have emphasised the need to accompany a test result with a confidence interval for the parameter that the hypothesis concerns. One approach to this was discussed in Chapter 4, where we used the MLE plus and minus 1.96 times the standard error determined by the information matrix (for a 95% confidence interval). More generally, as described earlier in this chapter, there is a correspondence between hypothesis tests and confidence intervals, so that a confidence interval can be determined corresponding to any particular test. This is obtained by identifying all values of θ_0 such that the null hypothesis would not be rejected. We start by illustrating this using the likelihood ratio and Wald tests, for the one-parameter hypothesis test that was the first of our testing problems considered in this extended example.

Based on the likelihood ratio and approximate Wald tests with estimated variance, the ranges of values for λ_0 that will not lead to rejection of the null hypothesis are:

$$\text{Likelihood ratio} \quad : \quad \left\{ \lambda_0 : 2\left[\ell(\hat{\lambda}) - \ell(\lambda_0)\right] < \chi^2_{1-\alpha}(1) \right\}$$

$$\text{Wald (approximate)} \quad : \quad \left\{ \lambda_0 : (\hat{\lambda} - \lambda_0)^2 I(\hat{\lambda}) < \chi^2_{1-\alpha}(1) \right\}.$$

For the data from group 1 analysed earlier in this section, these ranges correspond to the following 95% confidence intervals:

$$\text{Likelihood ratio} \quad : \quad \left\{ \lambda_0 : \ell(\lambda_0) > \ell(\hat{\lambda}) - 0.5\chi^2_{0.95}(1) \right\}$$
$$= \quad \left\{ \lambda_0 : \ell(\lambda_0) > -10.29 \right\} = \mathbf{(2.04, 3.02)}$$

$$\text{Wald (approximate)} \quad : \quad \left\{ \lambda_0 : |\hat{\lambda} - \lambda_0| < \sqrt{\chi^2_{0.95}(1)I(\hat{\lambda})^{-1}} \right\}$$
$$= \quad \left\{ \lambda_0 : |2.5 - \lambda_0| < 0.49 \right\} = \mathbf{(2.01, 2.99)}.$$

Notice that since $\sqrt{\chi^2_{1-\alpha}(1)} = z_{1-\alpha/2}$, the interval corresponding to the approximate Wald test is identical to that which would be obtained based on the usual method of confidence interval construction, that is, the MLE plus and minus 1.96 times the standard error. The interval based on the likelihood ratio test has the interpretation of including all parameter values that have sufficiently high likelihood, or in other words are sufficiently well supported by the data. Recalling that the approximate Wald test is equivalent to the score test in this example, it can be seen that the confidence intervals are consistent with the earlier *P*-values, in that the null hypothesis value of 3.0 is contained in the likelihood ratio interval but not in the approximate Wald test interval. For all practical purposes, however, these two intervals are essentially equivalent. Ideally the confidence interval should be calculated using whatever test has been used, however, in practice the approximate Wald test is the most common and convenient method for calculating a confidence interval for a single parameter.

The above test-based methods for one parameter can be generalised to calculate confidence regions for multiple parameters. To do this we use the same approach as above, based on the test statistics for testing hypotheses about all parameters, as described earlier in this chapter. For the likelihood ratio test this method again corresponds to the set of all parameter values that have sufficiently high likelihood. For our three parameter model, a 95% confidence region is the set of parameter values:

$$\left\{ (\lambda, \gamma_2, \gamma_3) : \ell(\lambda, \gamma_2, \gamma_3) > \ell(\hat{\lambda}, \hat{\gamma_2}, \hat{\gamma_3}) - 0.5\chi^2_{0.95}(3) \right\}$$
$$= \left\{ (\lambda, \gamma_2, \gamma_3) : \ell(\lambda, \gamma_2, \gamma_3) > -87.73 \right\}.$$

This set represents a three-dimensional region in which we are 95% confident that all three parameters lie. Strictly speaking, this means a confidence region calculated in this way will contain the true values of all three parameters in 95% of samples. Earlier we saw that the log-likelihood corresponding to the parameter combination $(\lambda, \gamma_2, \gamma_3) = (2.02, 1, 1)$ is -88.70. Since this does not exceed -87.73, this parameter combination would not be in the 95% confidence region, which is consistent with our earlier rejection of the null hypothesis $H_0 : \gamma_2 = 1$ and $\gamma_3 = 1$. Similarly the log-likelihood corresponding to all other parameter combinations can be used to determine those combinations that satisfy the required condition. The analogous method can also be used based on any of the other test statistics, although it is most intuitively meaningful based on the likelihood ratio test.

Finally, note that we have already discussed how to construct separate confidence intervals for multiple parameters in Chapter 4, based on the information matrix. However, the confidence region for all parameters will not simply correspond to the rectangle formed by these separate confidence intervals. For example, the 95% confidence region described above is plotted in Figure 6.4, for the parameters γ_2 and γ_3. In reality this region should be a three-dimensional "football" to accommodate λ, however, for simplicity a cross-section has been plotted at the value $\lambda = \hat{\lambda} = 2.5$. Figure 6.4 shows that the corners of the rectangle generated by the individual confidence intervals for γ_2 and γ_3 are not part of the confidence region. That is, although it is plausible that γ_2 or γ_3 could individually be at the extremes of their respective confidence interval ranges, it is not plausible that both parameters are simultaneously at the extremes of these ranges.

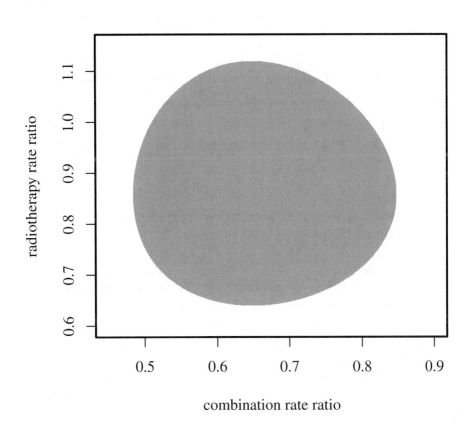

FIGURE 6.4
Cross-section of the three-dimensional 95% confidence region for $(\lambda, \gamma_2, \gamma_3)$, at the value $\lambda = 2.5$

Exercises

1. In the Chapter 5 exercises we considered the reduction in HIV viral load for each individual on antiviral therapy over a six month period. We considered a one-sample situation, in which for a group of individuals all on the same therapy we tested whether the average reduction was different to zero. A better study design is to include a control group receiving no treatment (or placebo) and to randomise patients to receive either no treatment or the antiviral treatment. We can then compare the average reduction in viral load in the two treatment groups. Let $(x_1, \ldots, x_n)$ be the observed reductions in viral load for individuals on no treatment, and let $(y_1, \ldots, y_n)$ be the reductions for individuals on antiviral therapy. Thus, there are equal numbers of individuals (n) on each treatment. We will assume that the reductions on no treatment have a $N(\mu, v)$ distribution, while the reductions on antiviral treatment have a $N(\mu + \delta, v)$ distribution. That is, μ denotes the mean reduction in the absence of treatment, and δ denotes the extra reduction received from the antiviral treatment. The hypotheses of interest in testing whether the antiviral treatment is effective at reducing viral load are:

$$H_0 : \delta = 0 \quad \text{versus} \quad H_1 : \delta \neq 0.$$

   (a) Write down the log-likelihood function in terms of the three parameters, $\ell(\mu, \delta, v)$. Derive the MLEs of each parameter.

   (b) Write down a standard error associated with $\hat{\delta}$. One way to do this is by using the information matrix, however, in this case you should be able to see from the form of $\hat{\delta}$ what the associated standard error is (which is easier than using the information matrix).

   (c) Construct the approximate Wald test for testing the above null hypothesis.

   (d) In this chapter we described how a Wald test based on a $\chi^2(1)$ distribution can be rewritten in terms of a standard normal distribution. Rewrite the approximate Wald test from part (c) in this way. How does this test differ from the usual two-sample t-test that could also be applied to this problem? In what circumstance will the two tests be equivalent?

2. In this exercise we consider a number of different tests associated with the disease prevalence in a particular population, based on a prevalence sample as considered in previous chapters. Based on these different tests we will also consider a number of different approaches to confidence interval calculation for the population prevalence (or in other words, for any binomial proportion). Begin by reviewing Exercise 1 from Chapter 4.

   (a) Write down the log-likelihood function for the population prevalence θ, as well as the MLE of θ and its standard error.

(b) Consider testing the hypothesis that the population prevalence is equal to a particular value:

$$H_0 : \theta = \theta_0 \quad \text{versus} \quad H_1 : \theta \neq \theta_0.$$

Write down the test statistics corresponding to each of the following tests: (i) likelihood ratio test; (ii) score test; (iii) Wald test; (iv) approximate Wald test. Show that using the score test is equivalent to using the Wald test.

(c) Suppose $\theta_0 = 0.5$, that is we wish to test whether the disease prevalence is equal to 50%. Evaluate each of the test statistics in part (b) (except the score test which is equivalent to the Wald test), based on the samples described in Example 3.2 from Chapter 3. Carry out each of these tests and give P-values.

(d) For the same data as used in part (c), plot the test statistics as a function of the null hypothesis value θ_0. By using the test-based definition of a confidence interval, mark a horizontal line on each graph, such that a 95% confidence interval corresponds to all θ_0 values that have a test statistic below this line. Hence calculate the 95% confidence interval corresponding to each test (you can use trial and error to work out where the function you have plotted crossed the horizontal line).

(e) Show that the confidence interval arising from the approximate Wald test in part (d) is equivalent to the usual confidence interval for a binomial proportion.

3. This question deals with multiple parameter tests for assessing the relationship between fertility and smoking exposure. Review Exercise 8 from Chapter 3, and Exercise 4 from Chapter 4, for the fertility study where mothers having smoking exposure have different fertility to mothers without such exposure. In those exercises we studied a likelihood function that was a function of two parameters, the fertility parameter for mothers with smoking history (p_2), and the relative fertility rate (γ). Start by writing down the log-likelihood function from Exercise 8(b) of Chapter 3. Our goal is to test the hypothesis that the fertility rates are identical, that is:

$$H_0 : \gamma = 1 \quad \text{versus} \quad H_1 : \gamma \neq 1.$$

(a) For the data set described in Exercise 7 of Chapter 3, evaluate the MLEs of p_2 and γ. Hence evaluate the maximum value achieved by the log-likelihood under the full model, $\ell(\hat{p}_2, \hat{\gamma})$.

(b) Write down the log-likelihood function under the assumption that the null hypothesis is true. Hence derive and evaluate the MLE of p_2 under the assumption that the null hypothesis is true and evaluate the maximum value achieved by the log-likelihood under the null model.

(c) Based on your results in parts (a) and (b), write down the likelihood ratio test statistic for testing the above hypotheses, and carry out a likelihood ratio test. Evaluate the P-value for this test.

(d) Using your results of Exercise 4(d) of Chapter 4, evaluate the approximate Wald test statistic for testing the above hypotheses. Carry out the test and calculate the *P*-value.

(e) Recall your results from parts (d) and (e) in Exercise 4 of Chapter 4. Explain why these are consistent with the tests conducted above.

4. Consider the stroke incidence study discussed in the extended examples of Chapters 3 and 4, and the examples throughout this chapter. In particular, we will assume that our sample (Y_1, Y_2) corresponds to the number of new cases of stroke in the high salt intake and low salt intake exposure groups, respectively. The observed sample is $(y_1, y_2) = (245, 239)$ based on a sample size of $(n_1, n_2) = (1150, 850)$ individuals having been followed for a total of $(F_1, F_2) = (5980, 3825)$ person years. The stroke incidence rates in the two groups are denoted by (λ_1, λ_2), with rate ratio $\gamma = \lambda_2/\lambda_1$, and the distribution of Y_i is Poisson$(\lambda_i F_i)$.

(a) As with the examples discussed in this chapter, assume first that the stroke rate is identical in the two diet groups, so that $\lambda_1 = \lambda_2 = \lambda$. Then the total number of strokes, $Y = Y_1 + Y_2$, has a Poisson(λF) distribution where $F = F_1 + F_2 = 9805$ person years. Recall the approach to simulation of this context used in the exercises of Chapter 1, using the function inc.sim described in Appendix 2. Simulate 10,000 studies under each of the assumptions $\lambda = 0.4, 0.5$ and 0.6. For each sample calculate the likelihood ratio and Wald test statistics for testing

$$H_0 : \lambda = 0.05 \quad \text{versus} \quad H_1 : \lambda \neq 0.05$$

and determine whether these statistics would lead to rejection of the null hypothesis. For each value of λ identify the proportion of repeated samples that lead to rejection of the null hypothesis and interpret your results. Hence comment on the relative merits of these two tests in this particular situation.

(b) Now consider the two-parameter model where we do not assume $\lambda_1 = \lambda_2$. Write down the log-likelihood function for the two-parameter model, $\ell(\lambda_1, \gamma)$. Making use of the MLEs and standard errors from the extended example of Chapter 4, conduct the likelihood ratio test of whether the stroke rates in the two diet groups are identical:

$$H_0 : \gamma = 1 \quad \text{versus} \quad H_1 : \gamma \neq 1.$$

5. Consider the number of heart attacks per week arriving at the emergency departments of two different hospitals. During one hundred different weeks the heart attack numbers arriving at each hospital were recorded. It was found that the sample means were $\bar{x} = 20$ heart attacks per week arriving at hospital 1 and $\bar{y} = 22$ heart attacks per week arriving at hospital 2. You can assume that the number of heart attacks in each week arriving at hospital 1 are independent and identically distributed with a Poisson distribution having mean λ_1. Likewise, you

can assume that the numbers of heart attacks in each week arriving at hospital 2 are independent and identically distributed with a Poisson distribution having mean λ_2, independently of hospital 1. In comparing the number of heart attacks arriving at the hospitals, it is of interest to test the hypothesis that the rates of arrival of heart attack patients are identical in the two hospitals.

(a) For the above setting write down the null hypothesis H_0 and the two-sided alternative hypothesis H_1, in terms of λ_1 and λ_2.

(b) Derive the maximum likelihood estimators of λ_1 and λ_2, first assuming H_0 and then assuming H_1. Calculate each of the corresponding maximum likelihood estimates for these data.

(c) Provide approximate standard errors associated with your estimates in part (b).

(d) Now consider a reparameterisation of the model in terms of the parameters θ_1 and θ_2, where $\theta_1 = \lambda_1 - \lambda_2$ and $\theta_2 = \lambda_2$. Repeat parts (a)–(c) in terms of θ_1 and θ_2, instead of λ_1 and λ_2.

(e) Derive the likelihood ratio test for testing H_0 versus H_1 and undertake the test for these data using a significance level of $\alpha = 0.01$.

(f) Repeat part (e) using an approximate Wald test and compare your conclusions from the two tests.

6. Consider the HIV viral load example in Exercise 1, based on a normal distribution model. Suppose that we now allow for the possibility that the variance in the control group (no treatment) is different from the variance in the antiviral treatment group. That is, we will now assume that the viral load reductions on no treatment have a $N(\mu, v_1)$ distribution, while the viral load reductions on antiviral treatment have a $N(\mu + \delta, v_2)$ distribution.

(a) First consider just the sample $(x_1, \ldots, x_n)$ of viral load reductions in the control group. For a given value v_0, derive the likelihood ratio test for testing $H_0 : v_1 = v_0$ versus $H_1 : v_1 \neq v_0$.

(b) Now consider the samples from both treatment groups, $(x_1, \ldots, x_n)$ and $(y_1, \ldots, y_n)$. Derive the likelihood ratio test for testing $H_0 : v_1 = v_2$ versus $H_1 : v_1 \neq v_2$.

(c) Find approximate critical regions for the tests in parts (a) and (b) assuming n is large and $\alpha = 0.05$.

7

Bayesian Inference

Most of this book has been concerned with the so-called frequentist approach to inference, which is based on the concept of repeated sampling and the relative frequency interpretation of probability. At a couple of points we have referred to the existence of a completely different approach, called the Bayesian approach. In one chapter we do not have enough space to give a full treatment of Bayesian inference, but given its growing importance in modern statistical practice we provide here an introduction. Our aim is to provide a grounding in the basic concepts of Bayesian statistics, supplemented by some simple illustrations based on our earlier examples and exercises. We first give a brief overview of how the Bayesian approach differs from the frequentist approach, including the subjective interpretation of probability, and then provide some basic technical details relating to Bayes' rule. Next we introduce the important Bayesian concepts of prior and posterior distributions, as well as the Bayesian counterpart of confidence intervals, credible intervals. The connection between Bayesian and likelihood inference is then reviewed, followed by a Bayesian re-examination of the treatment comparison example discussed in Chapter 5.

7.1 Probability and uncertainty

Bayesian inference is named after the Reverend Thomas Bayes, who discovered a probabilistic theorem in the eighteenth century that is now referred to as Bayes' rule. This theorem is the foundation of the Bayesian approach to statistical inference. Before moving on to discuss Bayes' rule and its importance, we begin by introducing some of the differences between Bayesian inference and the frequentist approach that we have used elsewhere in this book. In particular, we begin by contrasting the relative frequency definition of probability that underlies the repeated sampling interpretation of frequentist concepts such as confidence intervals and P-values, with an alternative view of probability that is used in Bayesian inference, namely, subjective probability.

The essence of the Bayesian approach is that it allows the data analyst to make inferences in terms of probability statements about the unknown parameters. This approach is quite different to the frequentist approach we have been discussing up until now, where the unknown parameters are considered to be fixed constants for which probability statements are not meaningful. To explore this further, consider the familiar concept of a confidence interval for the population prevalence, as was first introduced in Chapter 2. There we examined the simple statistical task of estimating the prevalence of disease using a sample of individuals from the population of interest. In this chapter we will examine this same example from a Bayesian point of view.

In Chapter 2 we used an illustrative example of a sample of 1000 individuals, 121 of whom have the disease. The estimated prevalence is therefore 12.1% with a standard error of 1.0% and a 95% confidence interval for the unknown population prevalence runs from 10.1% to 14.1%. We carefully considered the correct interpretation of this confidence interval in terms of coverage probability in repeated samples. That is, we regarded this interval estimate as a useful summary of uncertainty because it was calculated in such a way that 95% of such samples will produce a confidence interval that includes the true population prevalence.

This strict interpretation of a confidence interval, which requires us to think in terms of a large number of repeated samples, each with its own confidence interval, is one that some people find unintuitive. For this reason, the strict repeated sampling interpretation is often loosened to some extent when confidence intervals are used in practice. For example, it is not uncommon to summarise a confidence interval with a statement that we can be 95% confident that the unknown parameter lies somewhere in the range specified by the confidence interval. Although the term "confident" does not have a strict interpretation here, when one looks carefully at statements such as this, what is actually meant is that it is "likely" that the true parameter value lies in the calculated confidence interval. This is essentially an attempt to interpret the calculated confidence interval using a probability statement. However, as we know from our discussion in Chapter 2, such probability statements are not meaningful when they are made using a confidence interval calculated from a particular sample. Thus, for our prevalence example, it is not correct to say that there is a probability of 95% that the true prevalence lies between 10.1% and 14.1%. One of the main attractions of Bayesian inference is that it allows us to make this sort of probability statement in a meaningful way. But we shall see that this attractive feature does not come without a cost.

Recall the interpretation of probability that underlies the frequentist approach to inference, namely, that the probability of an event is the long-run relative frequency with which the event occurs in many repeated samples. Such an interpretation makes sense when our sampling process can be repeated, such as the tossing of a coin, but is more difficult to interpret when repeated sampling is not possible. For example, the interpretation of the statement "it will rain tomorrow with probability 80%" is not clear given that tomorrow cannot be repeated. Although it is possible to argue that the repeated sampling interpretation can be used by imagining what would happen in the hypothetical scenario that tomorrow could be repeated, some people find this interpretation somewhat cumbersome.

Bayesian inference, on the other hand, makes use of an alternative interpretation of probability, which is usually referred to as **subjective probability**. Under a subjective interpretation of probability, probability statements reflect the degree of belief that the person making the statement has that the event will occur. With this broader view of probability, statements such as "it will rain tomorrow with probability 80%" are just as meaningful as probability statements concerning contexts in which repeated sampling is possible. Indeed, under the subjective interpretation of probability used in Bayesian inference, probability statements can be made about anything that is uncertain. Thus, in Bayesian inference, probability statements are a quantification of **uncertainty**, rather than a quantification of what will occur in repeated samples.

This difference in interpretation leads to perhaps the most fundamental distinction between frequentist and Bayesian inference, namely, that Bayesian inference allows probability statements to be made about the parameters in a statistical model. Since parameters are simply constants whose values are unknown, Bayesian inference allows uncertainty about parameters to be expressed using subjective probability statements. This has some intuitive appeal, particularly given our discussion of the informal interpretation of confidence intervals earlier in this section. However, some statisticians argue that this comes at too high a cost in terms of subjectivity and assumptions that must be imposed on the analysis.

There have been many deep philosophical arguments about the meaning and applicability of probability, and it is beyond the scope of this book to attempt to resolve these disputes. Some further reading on foundational topics is provided in Appendix 3, particularly the book by Cox (2006) along with a number of other texts that discuss the foundations of probability and statistical inference. What we will do in this chapter, however, is to introduce some of the key concepts in Bayesian inference, since these concepts are becoming increasingly common in modern biostatistical practice.

7.2 Bayes' rule

The basic mechanism of Bayesian inference is the calculation of conditional probabilities. In Chapter 1, we reviewed the fact that if we consider two events A and B, the conditional probability that A occurs given that B has occurred, is defined as

$$\Pr(A \mid B) = \frac{\Pr(A \cap B)}{\Pr(B)},$$

where $\Pr(A \cap B)$ is the probability of both A and B occurring. The central tool of Bayesian inference, which we will call **Bayes' rule** but which is also known as **Bayes' theorem**, is the observation that if we consider the same definition of conditional probability in reverse, then it is clear that

$$\Pr(B \mid A) = \frac{\Pr(A \mid B)\Pr(B)}{\Pr(A)}.$$

Essentially then, Bayes' rule provides a mechanism for getting from a conditional probability that goes in one direction, A given B, to a conditional probability that goes in the reverse direction, B given A. For this reason, Bayes' rule and Bayesian inference was historically referred to as the method of **inverse probability**.

To understand how Bayes' rule is used in Bayesian inference, we need to take a broader interpretation of the events A and B, beyond what we mean by events in the context of frequentist probability. Firstly, we consider B to be a statement about the unknown parameter θ, so that Bayes' rule then involves probability statements about θ. As discussed in Section 7.1, this is acceptable using the subjective interpretation of probability in which such statements are interpreted as a quantification of our uncertainty about θ. Secondly, we consider A to be a statement about the observed sample, or the data, so that Bayes' rule then also involves probability statements about the data. These probability statements, which involve both conditional and unconditional probabilities, then form the basis for making Bayesian inferences about the parameter.

Specifically, we begin with a parametric model for how the data were generated, conditional on the parameter. This provides us with the $\Pr(A \mid B)$ part of Bayes' rule. Then we use Bayes' rule to invert the conditional probability to give us the $\Pr(B \mid A)$ part of Bayes' rule. This provides us with a probability distribution for the parameter, conditional on the data, and it is this probability distribution that is used as the basis of Bayesian inference. In the next section we will elaborate on these ideas and introduce some important terminology related to the above probability distributions, however, first we consider a simple example of the application of Bayes' rule.

Example 7.1 A common biostatistical application is diagnostic testing to determine the presence or absence of a particular disease. Consider a randomly sampled individual from a population in which the disease prevalence is q. We will assume that the prevalence q is known, or at least that we have a good estimate. We are interested in determining the disease status of the individual, which is unknown and will be denoted by θ. The individual's disease status can take just two values, which we will define to be

$$\theta = \begin{cases} 1 & \text{if disease is present} \\ 0 & \text{if disease is absent.} \end{cases}$$

The diagnostic test is carried out on the individual in order to obtain information about the disease status θ, which yields a test result that will be denoted by Y. The individual's test result can also take just two values, which we will define to be

$$Y = \begin{cases} 1 & \text{if the test result is positive} \\ 0 & \text{if the test result is negative.} \end{cases}$$

Suppose that we are only interested in deciding which value of θ is more likely, that is, whether it is more likely that the individual has the disease or does not have the disease. Prior to observing the individual's test result, our uncertainty about the disease status would be quantified using the disease prevalence in the population

$$\Pr(\theta = 1) = q \quad \text{and} \quad \Pr(\theta = 0) = 1 - q.$$

So if $q > (1-q)$, or equivalently $q > 0.5$, then our degree of belief in the disease status $\theta = 1$ is greater than our degree of belief in the disease status $\theta = 0$, and vice versa.

Now suppose that the individual's test result is positive, and consider how our uncertainty about the individual's disease status is modified by observing this test result. The extent to which our uncertainty about θ is modified by the observation that $Y = 1$ will depend on the accuracy of the diagnostic test. There are two probabilities that summarise the accuracy of a diagnostic test and hence influence our beliefs about θ. The first probability is the probability α of the test producing a false positive result, that is, producing a positive result for a person without the disease. The second probability is the probability β of the test producing a false negative result, that is, producing a negative result for a person with the disease. In view of their definitions, these measures of test accuracy are given by the conditional probabilities

$$\alpha = \Pr(Y = 1 \mid \theta = 0) \quad \text{and} \quad \beta = \Pr(Y = 0 \mid \theta = 1).$$

Obviously we would place more trust in the accuracy of the test result if α and β are small.

Bayes' rule can now be used to assess how our prior beliefs about θ have been modified by observing $Y = 1$. If we let q_1 and q_0 be the conditional probabilities that $\theta = 1$ and $\theta = 0$, respectively, given that we have observed a positive test result, then Bayes' rule implies

$$q_1 = \Pr(\theta = 1 \mid Y = 1) = \frac{\Pr(Y = 1 \mid \theta = 1)\Pr(\theta = 1)}{\Pr(Y = 1)} = \frac{(1-\beta)q}{\Pr(Y = 1)}$$

and

$$q_0 = \Pr(\theta = 0 \mid Y = 1) = \frac{\Pr(Y = 1 \mid \theta = 0)\Pr(\theta = 0)}{\Pr(Y = 1)} = \frac{\alpha(1-q)}{\Pr(Y = 1)}.$$

Thus, having observed the positive test result, our degree of belief in the disease status $\theta = 1$ is greater than our degree of belief in the disease status $\theta = 0$, if $q_1 > q_0$ or equivalently $q > \alpha/(1 + \alpha - \beta)$.

Some numerical calculations for particular values of α, β and q can illustrate the interpretation of these results. Suppose that the population of interest is a low prevalence population, say with $q = 0.05$. Then for any individual sampled at random from this population our prior belief would be strongly in favour of the individual not having the disease. Now consider two diagnostic tests, the first being quite accurate, with false positive and negative values of $\alpha = \beta = 0.01$, and the second being somewhat inaccurate, with $\alpha = \beta = 0.2$. For the accurate test $q > \alpha/(1 + \alpha - \beta) = 0.01$ so our belief would be modified in favour of the individual having the disease. For the inaccurate test $q < \alpha/(1 + \alpha - \beta) = 0.2$ so our belief would remain in favour of the individual not having the disease. The intuitive interpretation of this is that for a low prevalence population, a positive test result from an inaccurate test will not be convincing enough to modify our prior belief that the individual does not have the disease. On the other hand, if the test is accurate enough, then a positive test result will lead us to modify this belief.

Notice that since both q_1 and q_0 have $\Pr(Y = 1)$ in their denominators, the value of this probability was irrelevant for comparing q_1 and q_0 because it is simply a scaling factor that cancels out. However, if we actually wanted to calculate the value of q_1, rather than just compare it with q_0, then we would need to calculate $\Pr(Y = 1)$. This can be carried out by noticing that $q_0 + q_1 = 1$ because θ must be either 0 or 1, so that

$$\Pr(Y = 1) = (1 - \beta)q + \alpha(1 - q).$$

We shall see below that the denominator term in Bayes' rule plays the same sort of role more generally in Bayesian inference.

7.3 Prior and posterior distributions

We now elaborate on the use of Bayes' rule to provide an approach for conducting inferences about the parameter θ. The aim of a Bayesian analysis is to produce a probability distribution for the unknown θ that takes account of, or in other words conditions on, the information in the sample Y. This probability distribution quantifies the uncertainty in the parameter θ, conditional on having observed a particular value for the sample, $Y = y$. We will denote the distribution of θ given $Y = y$ by $p(\theta|y)$, which may be either a probability function if the parameter space is discrete, or a probability density function if the parameter space is continuous. Most parametric models in statistics are based on continuous parameter spaces so typically $p(\theta|y)$ will be a probability density function.

The notation $p(\theta|y)$ is an example of shorthand notation that will be used throughout this chapter to refer to a variety of distributions involving θ and Y. Thus, as is customary in describing the elements of Bayesian inference, we will use a general function p to stand for either a probability function or a probability density function, and the function arguments θ and y will tell us which distribution we are referring to. This was the case in defining $p(\theta|y)$ and will be the case for various other distributions described below.

Bayes' rule will be used to produce $p(\theta|y)$ by combining two fundamental quantities. The first is the distribution of the sample Y, given the parameter θ, which specifies the parametric model that we are assuming for the data. This may again be characterised by a probability function or a probability density function, depending on the type of sample Y, and in both cases the value of the function corresponding to an observation of $Y = y$ will be denoted by $p(y|\theta)$. The second is an assumed probability distribution for the parameter prior to the data having been observed. This distribution is characterised by the probability density function $p(\theta)$, assuming that θ can take values in a continuous parameter space. As for $p(\theta|y)$, in the less common situation that the parameter space is discrete, $p(\theta)$ is a probability function.

The combination of $p(\theta)$ and $p(y|\theta)$ to produce $p(\theta|y)$ is now facilitated by Bayes' rule. Re-expressing Bayes' rule from Section 7.2 using the notation from this section, we obtain

$$p(\theta|y) = \frac{p(y|\theta)p(\theta)}{p(y)} \propto p(y|\theta)p(\theta)$$

which is applicable regardless of whether the probability distributions are discrete or continuous. Notice that in addition to the three distributions $p(\theta)$, $p(y|\theta)$ and $p(\theta|y)$ discussed above, there is a fourth distribution $p(y)$ that occurs in the denominator of Bayes' rule. This is the distribution of the sample without conditioning on the parameter θ, called the **marginal distribution** of the sample Y. Since $p(y)$ does not depend on θ it will not affect the shape of our posterior distribution and only acts as a **normalising constant** which makes the probability distribution $p(\theta|y)$ a valid distribution that sums or integrates to 1.

The intuition behind using Bayes' rule in combination with a subjective interpretation of probability is as follows. The probability distribution specified by $p(\theta)$ quantifies our prior beliefs, or uncertainty, about the unknown parameter θ. We can then use the observed sample $Y = y$, to update our prior beliefs about θ. This is achieved by using Bayes' rule to produce a distribution that quantifies our updated beliefs about θ, $p(\theta|y)$. Leaving aside the normalising constant which is independent of θ, the form of Bayes' rule implies that this updated distribution is simply the product of the distribution quantifying our prior beliefs about the parameter, $p(\theta)$, and the distribution of the sample conditional on the parameter, $p(y|\theta)$.

In light of the above discussion, there are two very important pieces of terminology that are frequently used when describing a Bayesian analysis. Firstly, the distribution that quantifies our prior beliefs about the parameter, $p(\theta)$, is referred to as the **prior distribution**. Secondly, the distribution that quantifies our updated beliefs about the parameter after having observed the sample, $p(\theta|y)$, is referred to as the **posterior distribution**. The quantity $p(y|\theta)$, which is the link between the prior distribution and the posterior distribution, does not need any new terminology because it is simply the likelihood that we have discussed at length in other chapters. We will return to the role of the likelihood in Bayesian inference a number of times throughout this chapter.

Carrying out a Bayesian analysis is then seemingly simple: we just need to calculate the posterior distribution of θ using the ingredients described above. Based on this distribution, we can then make a variety of subjective probability statements that represent our beliefs about θ having observed the sample. For example, we can quote an interval within which θ lies with a certain probability, or we can give the probability that θ is greater than some value of special interest, such as 0 if θ measures the difference between two groups. While this sounds straightforward in principle, practical challenges arise due to two important complications.

Firstly, the computations involved in determining the posterior distribution are often very challenging. This is particularly the case for computations involving the marginal distribution $p(y)$ which may involve very difficult integrals. Example 7.2 illustrates this for a simple setting, but the problem magnifies greatly for very complex models. Fortunately, advances in Bayesian computational methods and software have greatly alleviated this complication, even for very complex models. Such methods are based on a class of simulation techniques called **Markov chain Monte Carlo** methods, which are discussed in detail in Bayesian inference texts such as Gelman et al. (2013).

Secondly, and more fundamentally, calculation of the posterior distribution requires two levels of assumptions, including an extra level over what is required for frequentist inference. The first level of assumptions is the model for the data given the parameter, $p(y|\theta)$, which is simply the likelihood function used in frequentist inference. This prominent role of the likelihood function in Bayesian inference is an important feature that we will return to later in the chapter. The second level of assumptions is the prior distribution for the parameter, $p(\theta)$. It is this component of Bayesian inference that is generally speaking the controversial one, since its presence tells us that conclusions about θ, in the form of the posterior distribution, cannot be obtained without making some prior assumptions about the unknown parameter. Some statisticians object to the use of Bayesian inference because of its perceived dependence on the prior distribution. This dependence may lead to concern that the results of an analysis will be determined by the prior assumptions rather than by the data being analysed. Other statisticians consider the specification of a prior distribution quite natural and find the ability to make probability statements about the parameter attractive. Either way, the prior distribution is the price we must pay in order to have the intuitively appealing interpretations associated with a Bayesian analysis.

Example 7.2 As an illustrative example we will work through some of the mechanics of Bayesian inference for a very simple example, the problem of assessing disease prevalence. Suppose that Y is the number of individuals who have a particular disease, out of a random sample of n individuals from a population of interest. The parameter is the population prevalence θ, which is the probability that a randomly chosen individual from the population will have the disease. The distribution of the sample Y, given a particular value for the parameter θ, can be specified using the binomial distribution

$$p(y|\theta) = \Pr(Y = y|\theta) \propto \theta^y (1-\theta)^{n-y}.$$

For now we have omitted the normalising constant $p(y)$, which is the denominator term in Bayes' rule that is constant with respect to θ. Later in this example we will briefly return to the normalising constant, which we also called the marginal distribution of Y.

Now let us consider our prior beliefs about θ, before considering the information contained in the sample. Suppose we had no prior information about θ, and that we therefore believed that there was no reason to give any value of θ more prior support than any other. We could represent this prior belief by giving θ a uniform prior distribution. In fact, this simply means specifying that

$$p(\theta) = 1 \qquad \text{for all } \theta \in [0,1].$$

Since the prior distribution is so simple in this case, it is straightforward to use Bayes' rule to calculate the posterior distribution of θ

$$p(\theta|y) \propto p(y|\theta)p(\theta) \propto \theta^y (1-\theta)^{n-y}.$$

With this step we have now turned the likelihood function for θ into a posterior distribution for θ. Thus, for this simple example where the likelihood function and the posterior distribution have the same form, frequentist and Bayesian inference will yield similar conclusions, albeit with different probabilistic interpretations. This, however, would not necessarily be the case for other prior distributions, as we will explore further later in the chapter.

Some examples of the posterior prevalence distribution for samples of size 10, 100, and 1000, are presented in Figure 7.1. Notice that the posterior distribution for the population prevalence has high probability density for values of θ that are close to the observed prevalence, y/n. Notice also that the range of θ values with high probability density is narrower when the sample size is larger. Furthermore, it can be seen that as the sample size gets larger, the posterior distribution seems to converge to a normal distribution. This asymptotic normality is a common feature of posterior distributions. All of these features of the posterior distribution are useful for making inferential statements about the population prevalence and we return to the manner in which we can use the posterior distribution later in this chapter.

It is worth noting in passing that the probability density functions plotted in Figure 7.1 required calculation of the normalising constant $p(y)$ in the denominator of the Bayes' rule calculation. This facilitates comparison between the different sample sizes depicted in Figure 7.1 because all of the probability densities integrate to 1 and are therefore comparable on the same scale. In this example, the requirement that $p(\theta|y)$ integrates to 1 leads to a normalising constant of the form

$$p(y) = \int_0^1 p(y|\theta)p(\theta)d\theta = \int_0^1 \theta^y(1-\theta)^{n-y}d\theta = B(y+1, n-y+1)$$

where B is a special mathematical function called the **beta function**. This function does not have a closed form so $p(y)$ requires numerical calculations using a computer, which is possible in many common statistical software packages. However, it should be remembered that although it was useful for our illustrative comparisons between different hypothetical samples, inclusion of the normalising constant in the posterior distribution calculation does not affect the shape of the posterior distribution, it only affects the scale of the y-axis in Figure 7.1.

7.4 Conjugate prior distributions

For a particular parametric model of the sample given the parameter, $p(y|\theta)$, the type of prior distribution that is chosen will determine the type of posterior distribution that is obtained. Since the posterior distribution will be used as the basis for our inferences about the parameter, there is some advantage to having a posterior distribution that is mathematically and computationally convenient to work with. This suggests that we could choose our prior distribution in such a way that we know the resulting posterior distribution will have a convenient form. We may go one step further, and

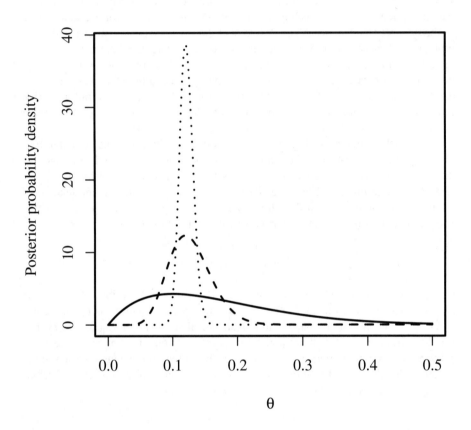

FIGURE 7.1
Posterior distribution of θ for three different prevalence samples: $y = 1$ diseased from a sample of $n = 10$ (solid line); $y = 12$ diseased from a sample of $n = 100$ (dashed line); and $y = 121$ diseased from a sample of $n = 1000$ (dotted line).

seek a prior distribution that leads to a posterior distribution that is in the same parametric family of probability distributions. When a particular type of prior distribution $p(\theta)$ leads to a posterior distribution $p(\theta|y)$ that has the same parametric form, then we call it a **conjugate prior distribution** for the model $p(y|\theta)$. Conjugate prior distributions are typically the most convenient and natural prior distributions, and are often the first choice that one considers in undertaking a Bayesian analysis.

A distribution may be a conjugate prior distribution for one model, but not for another model. That is, the property of being a conjugate prior distribution is a property that holds with respect to a particular parametric model for the sample. In a Bayesian analysis we often start by specifying a model for the sample that is aligned with how the sample was obtained, and then choose a prior distribution that is a conjugate prior for the particular model we have chosen.

A very important example of a conjugate prior distribution arises for parametric models in which $p(y|\theta)$ is a normal distribution with mean θ and known variance. For this model, if we choose a prior distribution $p(\theta)$ that is also a normal distribution, then the posterior distribution $p(\theta|y)$ will always be a normal distribution. In other words, the normal distribution is the conjugate prior distribution for a normal model where the parameter is the mean. Thus, the normal distribution can be thought of as being the conjugate prior distribution for itself, and so it is sometimes called **self-conjugate**. The normal model is such an important model in Bayesian inference that we will study it in some detail in the next section. Before doing this we return to the prevalence study discussed in Example 7.2, which will allow us to discuss the conjugate prior distribution for a binomial model.

Example 7.3 In Example 7.2 we considered a uniform prior distribution on the interval $[0,1]$ for the population prevalence θ. The uniform prior distribution is a specific case of a more general and flexible distribution on the interval $[0,1]$ called the beta distribution, denoted $\text{Beta}(\alpha,\beta)$. The beta distribution is commonly chosen as the prior distribution for the probability in a binomial distribution and leads to a prior distribution with two parameters $\alpha > 0$ and $\beta > 0$

$$p(\theta) = \frac{\theta^{\alpha-1}(1-\theta)^{\beta-1}}{B(\alpha,\beta)}$$

where B is the beta function that was discussed in Example 7.2. We can see that the uniform distribution is a special case of the beta distribution by setting $\alpha = \beta = 1$. However, as we will see in the exercises, the more general beta distribution allows much more flexibility in the shape of the distribution on the interval $[0,1]$.

Recall from Example 7.2 that the likelihood for the binomial prevalence model has the form

$$p(y|\theta) \propto \theta^y(1-\theta)^{n-y}.$$

It is therefore clear that the posterior distribution will have the same beta form that the prior distribution had. This is because, after dropping the term that does not depend on θ,

$$p(\theta|y) \propto p(y|\theta)p(\theta) \propto \theta^{y+\alpha-1}(1-\theta)^{n-y+\beta-1}.$$

In other words, if we assume a Beta(α, β) prior distribution then the posterior distribution is Beta$(y + \alpha, n - y + \beta)$, having observed y individuals with the disease out of a sample of n individuals. We have therefore shown that the conjugate prior distribution for the probability in a binomial model is the beta distribution. A useful way of thinking about the Beta(α, β) prior distribution is that it is analogous to assuming prior knowledge of a similar strength to having $\alpha - 1$ additional individuals with the disease and $\beta - 1$ additional individuals without the disease. This can be seen by comparing the form of $p(y|\theta)$ and $p(\theta|y)$.

7.5 Inference for a normal mean

Although the mechanics of the binomial model with a beta prior distribution make a nice introduction to Bayesian analysis, the overwhelmingly most important application of Bayesian inference relates to normal distributions. This is not because most quantities of interest follow a normal distribution, but rather because so many summary statistics and estimators of important parameters have normal sampling distributions, at least in large samples. In the extended example discussed in Section 7.10 we will explore these issues further, and show how Bayesian inference based on normal distributions can be applied in situations where the outcome is essentially non-normal. In this section, however, we will concentrate on the basic calculations of Bayesian inference for normal models, in particular focussing on inference for the mean of a normal distribution.

7.5.1 Single observation

Suppose we have a single random variable Y that follows a normal distribution with unknown mean θ and known variance σ^2. The assumption of known variance is of course unrealistic, but it enables us to work through some of the basic details in a simple case. Furthermore, there is a very real sense in which variance estimation is usually of secondary concern, and variance estimates can often be "plugged in" if the main aim is estimation of the mean. The sampling model can be represented by the normal density function

$$p(y|\theta) = \frac{1}{\sigma\sqrt{2\pi}} \exp\left\{-\frac{1}{2\sigma^2}(y - \theta)^2\right\}.$$

Although the normal density function may look formidable, its key feature is that it is an exponential of a quadratic function of θ. It follows that the conjugate prior density function is also the exponential of a quadratic function of θ, because only then will the product $p(y|\theta)p(\theta)$ remain the exponential of a quadratic function of θ. Thus, the conjugate prior density function has the form

$$p(\theta) = \exp\left\{A(\theta - B)^2 + C\right\} \propto \exp\left\{A(\theta - B)^2\right\}$$

which can be rewritten as

$$p(\theta) \propto \exp\left\{-\frac{1}{2\tau_0^2}(\theta - \mu_0)^2\right\}$$

using the reparameterisation $\tau_0^2 = -(2A)^{-1}$ and $\mu_0 = B$. That is, the conjugate prior density function has the form of a normal distribution, $N(\mu_0, \tau_0^2)$. We can therefore add to the long list of interesting properties of the normal distribution that a conjugate prior for the mean of a normal distribution is itself a normal distribution. This is what we meant in Section 7.4 when we said that the normal distribution is self-conjugate.

With this conjugate prior distribution, we can now consider the posterior distribution of θ. Combining the likelihood and the prior using Bayes' rule, and ignoring factors that are constant with respect to the parameter θ, we obtain

$$p(\theta|y) \propto p(y|\theta)p(\theta)$$

$$\propto \exp\left\{-\frac{1}{2}\left[\frac{(y-\theta)^2}{\sigma^2} + \frac{(\theta - \mu_0)^2}{\tau_0^2}\right]\right\}.$$

Some algebra can then be used to express this as

$$p(\theta|y) \propto \exp\left\{-\frac{(\theta - \mu_1)^2}{2\tau_1^2}\right\}$$

where

$$\mu_1 = \frac{(\mu_0/\tau_0^2) + (y/\sigma^2)}{(1/\tau_0^2) + (1/\sigma^2)} \quad \text{and} \quad \frac{1}{\tau_1^2} = \frac{1}{\tau_0^2} + \frac{1}{\sigma^2}.$$

This means that the posterior distribution is $N(\mu_1, \tau_1^2)$.

The form of the posterior distribution leads to a number of important observations. Firstly, in manipulating normal distributions, the inverse of the variance plays a prominent role, and is called the **precision**. The algebra above shows that for normal data with a normal prior distribution, the posterior precision equals the prior precision plus the data precision. In other words, the uncertainty represented by the spread of the posterior distribution is a combination of uncertainty due to the prior distribution and variability in the data. This means that if either component is reduced, the posterior uncertainty reduces. Furthermore, we can see that the posterior mean is a weighted average of the prior mean and the data, with the weights being proportional to the precision of the prior distribution and the data, respectively. This provides a nice illustration of the manner in which the prior distribution and the data combine to produce the posterior distribution.

7.5.2 Multiple observations

It is straightforward to extend the above discussion based on a single observation to the situation where we have a sample of independent and identically distributed observations, $Y = (Y_1, \ldots, Y_n)$. The likelihood function for the mean θ, based on the observed value of a sample of n observations $Y = y$, depends only on the observed value of the sufficient statistic $\overline{Y} = \overline{y}$, the observed value of the sample mean. Using our shorthand notation we can therefore write

$$p(y|\theta) = L(\theta;y) = \prod_{i=1}^{n} p(y_i|\theta) \propto p(\overline{y}|\theta)$$

where the last distribution refers to the normal distribution of the sample mean with known variance $N(\theta, \sigma^2/n)$. Using our results for the single normal observation we can then see that the posterior density $p(\theta|y) = p(\theta|\overline{y})$ is the density function from a $N(\mu_n, \tau_n^2)$ distribution, where

$$\mu_n = \frac{\mu_0(1/\tau_0^2) + \overline{y}(n/\sigma^2)}{(1/\tau_0^2) + (n/\sigma^2)} \qquad \text{and} \qquad \frac{1}{\tau_n^2} = \frac{1}{\tau_0^2} + \frac{n}{\sigma^2}.$$

These formulae are very instructive. Firstly, they are a natural generalisation of the corresponding formulae for the single observation case. Thus, we can see that the posterior precision $1/\tau_n^2$ is the sum of the prior precision $1/\tau_0^2$ and the data precision n/σ^2. Likewise, the posterior mean μ_n is a weighted average of the prior mean μ_0 and the sample mean $\overline{y}$, weighted by the prior precision and the data precision, respectively. This means that if the sample size is large, so that the data precision is large, then the posterior distribution will be primarily determined by the sample mean $\overline{y}$ and the variance σ^2. It also gives us some intuition about how the information from the prior distribution is incorporated into the posterior distribution. For example, if the prior variance τ^2 is similar in magnitude to the sampling variance σ^2 then the prior distribution has the same weight as one extra observation with the value μ_0. Furthermore, if the prior variance becomes larger with n remaining fixed, or if n becomes larger with the prior variance remaining fixed, the posterior distribution approaches a form that is completely independent of the prior specification, namely, $N(\overline{y}, \sigma^2/n)$. This shows us that when the information in the sample greatly outweighs the information in the prior distribution then the posterior distribution is essentially unaffected by the prior specification.

The normal mean model discussed in this section is instructive because it transparently shows how the prior and the likelihood combine to produce the posterior distribution. Although other models do not always have formulae that are as interpretable as the model discussed in this section, the concept remains basically the same: the posterior distribution can be thought of as an average of the prior and the likelihood. In its entirety the posterior distribution quantifies the overall uncertainty in the parameter after combining the information contained in the prior and the likelihood. In the next section we will consider how specific features of the posterior distribution can be used to produce counterparts to the point and interval estimates discussed previously for frequentist inference.

7.6   Point and interval estimation

The fundamental object of Bayesian inference is the posterior distribution, and the overarching philosophy is to use the entire posterior distribution as a summary of our uncertainty about the parameter. Nonetheless, having obtained a posterior distribution, practical considerations often make it desirable to use the posterior distribution to produce point and interval estimates of the parameter. Essentially, this amounts to choosing certain key features of the posterior distribution to summarise our beliefs about the parameter, having observed the sample. In this section we will consider how this can be done, focussing on our previous normal and binomial models as illustrations.

In our discussion of estimation concepts in Chapter 2 we referred to a point estimate as a single best value with which to estimate the unknown parameter θ. In a Bayesian context, a point estimate is a single value of θ that best summarises the posterior distribution. Unfortunately, the definition of "best" is not unique, so there is more than one way to use the posterior distribution to produce a point estimate. One common method is to use the mode of the posterior distribution, that is, the value of θ for which the posterior probability density function is maximised. This estimate is called the **maximum posterior estimate** or sometimes more elaborately the **maximum a posteriori estimate**. Such an estimate is often considered intuitively appealing since it can loosely be interpreted as the most probable value of the unknown parameter according to the posterior distribution. It can also be considered the Bayesian version of the frequentist MLE, which is the most supported parameter value according to the likelihood function. An alternative approach to Bayesian point estimation is to use the mean of the posterior distribution, or indeed other measures of central tendency such as the median. For the normal mean model the posterior distribution is a normal distribution which is always symmetric and unimodal, so these different methods of estimation will all lead to the same value, namely, μ_n defined in Section 7.5.2. However, this will not always be the case, as illustrated below in Example 7.4.

A natural extension of point estimation using the maximum posterior estimate is an interval estimate constructed by finding an interval with high probability under the posterior distribution. The definition of "high" in this case is usually taken to be 95%, but could also be some other appropriate value such as 90% or 99%. Such an interval is called a **credible interval**, and can be considered the Bayesian version of a confidence interval. A 95% credible interval has the interpretation that there is a probability of 95% that the unknown parameter value lies within the interval. As discussed in Section 7.1, this is a highly appealing interpretation, and is one the people often wrongly ascribe to the frequentist confidence interval.

Although the interpretation of a credible interval is intuitively appealing, a technical complexity arises in that there is not just one interval that has 95% posterior probability. This means that a further requirement is needed to define such an interval estimate in a unique way. The requirement that is usually used is that the interval of values must not only contain 95% posterior probability, but must also be constructed such that no value outside the interval has higher posterior density than the values inside the interval. In this way the credible interval is uniquely defined as the **highest posterior density interval**.

Recall that for the normal mean model discussed in Section 7.5.2, the posterior distribution is the $\mathrm{N}(\mu_n, \tau_n^2)$ distribution. In this case the 95% credible interval for the mean θ will be the symmetric interval $\mu_n \pm 1.96\tau_n$, which is centred around the maximum posterior estimate μ_n. It is interesting to consider how this interval behaves when the prior distribution is not very informative relative to the sample. In Section 7.5.2, we discussed what happens to the posterior distribution in this case, which is that it approaches a form that is completely independent of the prior specification, namely, $\mathrm{N}(\bar{y}, \sigma^2/n)$. That is, $\mu_n \approx \bar{y}$ and $\tau_n^2 \approx \sigma^2/n$, so that the 95% credible interval reduces to $\bar{y} \pm 1.96\sigma/\sqrt{n}$. Remarkably, this is precisely the same interval that we would use as a 95% confidence interval. In other words, when the prior is not very informative compared to the sample, then the Bayesian point and interval estimates are approximately the same as the frequentist point and interval estimates. In both cases, all of the information about θ is obtained from the sample, or equivalently the likelihood. The concept of a prior distribution that is not very informative compared to the sample is an important concept that will be taken up in the next section, but first we will explore how the estimation concepts discussed in the current section carry over to another model, the binomial prevalence model.

Example 7.4 In a prevalence sample where y individuals have the disease out of n individuals, we saw in Example 7.3 that the posterior distribution for the population prevalence θ is $\mathrm{Beta}(y+\alpha, n-y+\beta)$, assuming we started with a $\mathrm{Beta}(\alpha, \beta)$ prior distribution. Point estimates based on the posterior distribution can be derived using the properties of the beta distribution, as described in Appendix 1. In particular, the maximum posterior estimate of θ is the mode of the beta posterior distribution. Assuming we have at least one diseased and one non-diseased individual in the sample, so that both $y + \alpha > 1$ and $n - y + \beta > 1$, then the mode is

$$\hat{\theta} = \frac{y+\alpha-1}{(n-y+\beta-1)+(y+\alpha-1)} = \frac{y+\alpha-1}{n+\alpha+\beta-2}.$$

Notice that if we assume a uniform prior with $\alpha = \beta = 1$, then $\hat{\theta}$ is identical to the MLE y/n. In this case, assuming a large sample size, the normal approximation to the beta distribution gives

$$\theta \mid y \overset{d}{\approx} \mathrm{N}\left(\hat{\theta}, \frac{\hat{\theta}(1-\hat{\theta})}{n}\right).$$

This leads to the 95% credible interval for θ

$$\hat{\theta} \pm 1.96\sqrt{\hat{\theta}(1-\hat{\theta})/n}$$

which is equivalent to the 95% confidence interval that we obtained based on the

MLE in Example 2.5 of Chapter 2. We also discussed alternative methods for constructing a Bayesian point estimate, particularly the mean of the posterior distribution. Using the mean of a beta distribution we obtain the estimate

$$\tilde{\theta} = \frac{y + \alpha}{n + \alpha + \beta}$$

which, in the case of a uniform prior, becomes $(y+1)/(n+2)$. Notice that, unlike the maximum posterior estimate, the mean of the posterior distribution is not equivalent to the MLE when we assume a uniform prior distribution, but it will be approximately equivalent to the MLE in large samples.

7.7 Non-informative prior distributions

The concordance between the Bayesian credible interval and the frequentist confidence interval discussed in the previous section arises because of our assumed prior distribution which was essentially "non-informative" relative to the information in the likelihood. The same sort of result can often arise in practical Bayesian analysis, in the sense that the inference we arrive at is often not affected substantially by the specified prior distribution. This leads to the question: how do we know when the prior distribution will be non-informative? A general answer to this question is somewhat complex and beyond our scope here, but we can consider it for the normal mean model and binomial prevalence model that we have been discussing in this chapter. In particular, for the one-sample normal mean model with known variance, it is not hard to work out just how informative any particular prior distribution will be. Indeed, we have already seen that a prior with similar variance to the sampling variance will have similar weight to one additional observation in the sample. Similarly, in the prevalence estimation problem, we saw in Example 7.3 that one way of thinking about the parameters of the conjugate beta prior distribution was in terms of additional observations. Both of these results allow us to assess the informativeness of a particular prior distribution relative to the informativeness of additional observations in the sample. While this is useful for these specific models, for other models this may not be possible, particularly where a conjugate prior may be less appropriate. In such cases it may be necessary to experiment a little with the prior specification to gain some appreciation of how influential it may be.

The concept of a **non-informative prior distribution** is one that has received a lot of attention in Bayesian statistics. Some people have argued that it is best to use a non-informative prior distribution because this allows the data to "speak for themselves", and limits the danger of letting subjective prior opinions unduly influence the final results. Others have taken the view that this is something of a misconception, because if we can make a reasonable range of alternative assumptions about the prior distribution and they result in a wide range of different conclusions, then it is most likely the case that the data themselves do not contain a very clear message about the parameter. This sensitivity to the prior distribution may be considered important information in some contexts. Nonetheless, for practical purposes where we have a reasonably large amount of data and a small number of parameters, then the notion of a non-informative prior distribution can be a useful starting point for a Bayesian analysis.

The precise nature of an appropriate non-informative prior distribution depends on the model. For the normal mean model, it is clear that a non-informative prior distribution arises by allowing the variance of the prior for the mean θ to be very large. Indeed, according to our previous discussion, the larger the variance is, the less informative the prior becomes relative to observations in the sample. A convenient way of representing a non-informative prior in this case is to say that the prior density for the mean θ is uniform on the whole real line $(-\infty, \infty)$. That is,

$$p(\theta) \propto 1 \qquad \text{for all } \theta \in (-\infty, \infty).$$

This is somewhat similar to the way we used a uniform distribution as a non-informative prior distribution for the binomial prevalence sample in Example 7.2. However, an important distinction is that for the normal mean model, the uniform prior is an example of what is called an **improper prior distribution**, because it is of course not possible to have a distribution giving positive probability to all finite segments of the whole real line. The total probability would then be infinite, not 1 as it must be for a proper probability distribution. Fortunately, because the likelihood function is itself a normal density when regarded as a function of θ, the posterior distribution is perfectly proper despite the improper prior. We can therefore regard the improper prior specification as a convenient approximation to a very "flat" proper prior density, and use the posterior distribution in the same way as if the prior had been a proper distribution.

In other models, the notion of a non-informative prior distribution becomes a little more complex, and the uniform distribution is not always the natural choice. We will not pursue this issue further here, but it is taken up in greater detail by more advanced Bayesian inference texts, such as the book by Carlin and Louis (2000) and further texts discussed in Appendix 3.

7.8   Multiple parameters

In principle, our introduction to prior and posterior distributions in Section 7.3 applies to both single parameter models and multiple parameter models where θ is a vector, $\theta = (\theta_1, \ldots, \theta_p)$. The multiple parameter situation is of course more complex, since the prior and posterior distributions will then be multivariate distributions, but conceptually the interpretation is the same as in the single parameter case. In particular, the multivariate prior and posterior probability distributions quantify our uncertainty about the collection of parameters $\theta = (\theta_1, \ldots, \theta_p)$, before and after our sample is observed. Furthermore, key features of the multivariate posterior distribution can be used for estimation purposes, as was discussed for the one-dimensional case in Section 7.6. Thus, for example, it is possible to construct a **credible region** for a parameter vector, which is a generalisation of the credible interval discussed in Section 7.6. This is a Bayesian analogue of the confidence region that we introduced in Section 6.10 from a frequentist perspective.

In fact, the Bayesian approach is often seen as advantageous in multiple parameter situations, by virtue of the fact that the parameters in the model are viewed as having a probability distribution. This means that in very high-dimensional models we can tie together a collection of the parameters using the assumption that each parameter in the collection has the same probability distribution. For example, if we wish to estimate a collection of means, such as the mean cholesterol level in each of a number of local areas, then we may be able to model the collection of means as if they came from a common probability distribution. Here, the mean of the common distribution would represent the overall mean-of-means and the variance would represent the extent of variability between the areas. This approach, and more complex variants of this approach, often allow convenient model specification and inference for high-dimensional contexts because the common probability model for the collection of parameters introduces greater parsimony into the model and makes the model parameters more easily estimable. Such models, which are sometimes referred to as **hierarchical models** or **multilevel models**, are often useful in biostatistics and are a core tool in Bayesian data analysis, as exemplified in the the book by Gelman et al. (2013).

One property of multiple parameter models that we discussed for frequentist inference and which is also important in Bayesian inference is that they may contain nuisance parameters. We introduced the concept of a nuisance parameter in Chapter 3, where we saw that it is a parameter that occurs in our model but which is not of any interest in it own right. The extended examples of Chapters 3 and 4 considered an important context in which nuisance parameters occur, namely, where the difference in disease rates between two groups is of interest but where the actual disease rates in each group are of less interest. Another very important context in which nuisance parameters can occur is where the mean in a normal model is of interest but the variance is not. Since we considered Bayesian inference for a normal mean in some depth when the variance is known, we will briefly consider how this generalises to the situation where the variance is unknown and is a nuisance parameter in the model.

Firstly, consider how a nuisance variance parameter is dealt with in frequentist inference for a normal mean. It can be shown that the MLE of a normal mean with unknown variance is always the sample mean, regardless of the value of the unknown variance. Thus, the nuisance parameter does not affect point estimation of the parameter of interest in this context. However, the sampling distribution of the MLE is dependent on the unknown variance, so the nuisance parameter will affect frequentist inferences based on the MLE. The usual approach to dealing with this is to use the sample variance S_{n-1}^2 as an estimator of the unknown variance σ^2, and to base our inferences about the mean θ on the t-distribution with $n-1$ degrees of freedom, using the fundamental property

$$\frac{\overline{Y} - \theta}{S_{n-1}/\sqrt{n}} \stackrel{d}{=} t_{n-1}.$$

Remember, from a frequentist point of view, this is the distribution of a random variable observable in the sample, given a specific value for the parameter θ.

It turns our that the Bayesian and frequentist approaches to this problem have a remarkable convergence in the situation where we choose a non-informative prior distribution. In particular, it turns out that the Bayesian posterior distribution for the mean, under a non-informative prior distribution, is the same t-distribution

$$\frac{\theta - \overline{y}}{s_{n-1}/\sqrt{n}} \,\Big|\, \{\overline{Y} = \overline{y},\ S_{n-1} = s_{n-1}\} \stackrel{d}{=} t_{n-1}.$$

In this case, however, we have a distribution for the parameter θ, conditional on the observed values of the sufficient statistics $\overline{Y} = \overline{y}$ and $S_{n-1} = s_{n-1}$. Thus, in the same way as for the simpler known-variance calculation, Bayesian credible intervals are just the same as standard frequentist confidence intervals. In this case the Bayesian approach has an intuitive interpretation. In particular, since the posterior t-distribution is more spread out than the corresponding normal distribution based on the same standard error, the posterior distribution can be thought of as allowing for the additional uncertainty introduced by the fact that the variance is estimated from the data rather than being known. This means that Bayesian probability statements quantifying the uncertainty in θ will reflect the additional uncertainty that arises from not knowing the value of the nuisance variance parameter.

7.9   Connection to likelihood inference

In previous sections we have seen some specific instances in which the Bayesian and frequentist approaches lead to similar inferences when the prior is non-informative. We now consider how the Bayesian concepts of this chapter tie in more generally with the likelihood concepts that underlie our discussion of frequentist inference elsewhere in this book. In fact, likelihood is a fundamental unifying concept between the Bayesian and frequentist approaches. We have already seen in this chapter that the likelihood function plays a central role in Bayesian inference. In this section we see how it can be used to draw a connection between frequentist inference based on maximum likelihood estimation and Bayesian inference with a non-informative prior distribution.

In Chapter 4 we discussed the fact that, in large samples, the sampling distribution of the MLE is approximately multivariate normal with mean equal to the parameter vector θ and variance-covariance matrix equal to the inverse of the information matrix $I(\theta)$. This is a frequentist statement about the sampling distribution of the estimator $\hat{\Theta}$ given a fixed value for the parameter θ, which can be written as

$$\hat{\Theta} \mid \theta \stackrel{d}{\approx} N\big(\theta, I(\theta)^{-1}\big).$$

Now suppose that the variance appearing in this result can be precisely enough estimated that we can think of it as essentially known. Then our discussion of Bayesian inference for a normal mean with known variance can be used to turn the above result around so that we obtain an approximate posterior distribution for θ. In particular, under a non-informative prior distribution, the posterior distribution is obtained by multiplying the likelihood by a constant, which in this case therefore leads to the approximate posterior distribution

$$\theta \mid \{\hat{\Theta} = \hat{\theta}\} \stackrel{d}{\approx} N\big(\hat{\theta}, I(\hat{\theta})^{-1}\big).$$

Since the MLE is a sufficient statistic for θ this is equivalent to a posterior distribution given the observed data $Y = y$

$$\theta \mid \{Y = y\} \stackrel{d}{\approx} N\big(\hat{\theta}, I(\hat{\theta})^{-1}\big).$$

The above discussion implies that, assuming we use a non-informative prior distribution and have a sufficiently large sample, the Bayesian posterior distribution for the parameter θ is an approximation to the frequentist sampling distribution for the MLE of θ. The practical implication of this observation is that frequentist inferential summaries, such as the MLE and a 95% confidence interval, will be similar to Bayesian inferential summaries, such as the mode of the posterior distribution and a 95% credible interval. This draws a connection between large sample Bayesian inference using a non-informative prior and large sample frequentist inference using the likelihood function. Of course, when an informative prior is used then the Bayesian analysis will no longer necessarily be similar to the likelihood analysis. In this case the Bayesian analysis becomes a weighted average of our prior beliefs and the information contained in the likelihood function, whereas the frequentist analysis is based solely on information contained in the likelihood function.

7.10 Extended example

The objective of this extended example is to illustrate the use of Bayesian inference for a common standard analysis, namely, the comparison of two proportions in a binomial model. We will re-examine the extended example on response to treatment for HIV that was introduced in Chapter 5. As well as demonstrating the basic concepts of Bayesian inference, including the calculation of prior and posterior distributions, this example allows further exploration of the similarities and differences between the Bayesian and frequentist approaches to inference. An important difference from the frequentist analysis is that the Bayesian analysis will not place great emphasis on hypothesis testing. Instead, we will focus on using the posterior distribution as an overall summary of our uncertainty about the difference between the two treatment groups, and investigating the impact that our choice of prior distribution has on the analysis.

7.10.1 Randomised trial

Recall the extended example from Chapter 5, in which we considered a trial of two antiviral treatments for individuals who are HIV positive. The results were summarised in Table 5.2. The first treatment was a standard or control therapy, involving a single drug, while the second treatment involved administering the control therapy in combination with a second drug. Participants were randomised to the two groups, and the "response" to treatment was the binary indicator of whether or not viral load was adequately reduced at the end of a six-month period of treatment.

As previously, we will focus on comparing the so-called response rates by examining their difference. In particular, our primary focus will be on making inferences about the difference in population response rates, using information from the sample responses and various assumed prior distributions.

7.10.2 Model

We will again use the two sample binomial model for the data. We subscript quantities associated with the control therapy with a 0 and the combination therapy with a 1. The number of individuals on each therapy is $n_0 = n_1 = n/2$, where n is the total number of individuals in the study. Since we will base the analysis on a binomial model for the number showing a positive response on each therapy, the full data vector of binary responses y can be reduced to the sufficient statistics x_0 and x_1, the numbers achieving a response on the two therapies, respectively. There are two parameters in the model, p_0 and p_1, the population response rates for each therapy. Assuming independence of the outcome from each individual, the model assumes that x_0 and x_1 are the observed values of random variables with $\text{Bin}(n_0, p_0)$ and $\text{Bin}(n_1, p_1)$ distributions, respectively.

The model contains two parameters but we are really only interested in a comparison between them, so it is useful to focus the analysis on a parameter that represents this comparison. We will use the difference between the two parameters, $\theta = p_1 - p_0$, which is called the risk difference. Although we will not study them in this example, other comparative parameters could also have been used, including the risk ratio or relative risk, p_1/p_0, and the odds ratio, $[p_1/(1-p_1)]/[p_0/(1-p_0)]$.

With the comparative measure θ as our parameter of interest, the other parameter in the model, which can be chosen to be either p_0 or p_1, becomes a nuisance parameter. Typically, the nuisance parameter would be taken to be the control rate, p_0. Inference for θ then means that we are implicitly transforming our parameter space of interest from "all possible values of p_0 and p_1" to "all possible values of θ and the nuisance parameter p_0". In fact, for an approximate Bayesian analysis that is adequate for our purposes, it will be possible to completely ignore the nuisance parameter, p_0.

Recall from the extended example in Chapter 5 that we focussed attention on the sample response rates $\hat{p}_0 = x_0/n_0$ and $\hat{p}_1 = x_1/n_1$, as estimates of the unknown p_0 and p_1. We also used the sample response rate difference $\hat{\theta} = \hat{p}_1 - \hat{p}_0$ as an estimate for the true difference θ. In calculating a confidence interval for θ based on $\hat{\theta}$, we implicitly used the fact that with reasonable sample size then $\hat{\theta}$ is an observation from a sampling distribution that is approximately normal with mean θ and variance $p_1(1-p_1)/n_1 + p_0(1-p_0)/n_0$. To obtain a confidence interval we substituted the estimates $\hat{p}_0$ and $\hat{p}_1$ for the true values p_0 and p_1 in this variance expression. These standard results can now be used in a Bayesian framework, by observing that we are assuming that $\hat{\theta}$ is an observation from an approximate normal distribution $\mathrm{N}(\theta, 0.004942)$, after substituting the values $\hat{p}_0 = 0.47$ and $\hat{p}_1 = 0.57$ into the variance. This normal model is precisely the "normal mean with known variance" model that we introduced in Section 7.5.

In the view of the above model, the remainder of this extended example will discuss how to use our results from Section 7.5 to make Bayesian inferences about the treatment difference parameter θ. Before doing so, however, we recap on three important assumptions and approximations that we have made in developing our model:

1. We have ignored the nuisance parameter, assuming that inference about the difference between response rates can be made independently of the actual rates;

2. We have assumed that the variance is known, although in fact we are plugging in an empirical estimate from the data;

3. We have assumed that the sample size is large enough that the normal distribution provides an adequate approximation to the sampling distribution for the difference between two binomial proportions.

A more complete Bayesian analysis would investigate the sensitivity of conclusions to possible inaccuracies in these assumptions. For example, there might be particular concerns with these assumptions if the sample sizes were small or the event rates were close to zero or 100%. However, given the sample sizes in this example are reasonably large and the observed event rates are well away from zero and 100%, we would expect the method to behave reasonably, and the calculations presented below provide an illustration of a basic analysis method that is widely applicable.

7.10.3 Prior distributions

To proceed with the Bayesian analysis, we need to specify a prior distribution for θ. The convenient choice is a normal distribution, because of the conjugate distribution property that we discussed earlier in the chapter. We therefore assume the prior distribution

$$\theta \overset{d}{=} \mathrm{N}(\mu, \tau^2).$$

To a large extent the choice of a normal distribution to represent prior beliefs in this case is not a strong assumption. The critical issue is the choice of the prior mean and variance. We will consider three possible choices. The first is the non-informative prior that we have already considered in Section 7.7, and which in the present context represents the belief that there is no reason to give greater support to any particular value of the treatment group difference compared to any other value. The other two choices of prior distribution will be called the "sceptical" and "enthusiastic" prior distributions.

The sceptical prior distribution represents the beliefs of a sceptic who is doubt-ful that the new combination therapy is really likely to produce worthwhile benefits. There are many possible ways of formalising such a sceptical view, but one reason-able approach is to specify a prior distribution that has a mean of zero, corresponding to no benefit, while allowing a small prior probability, say 5%, that the difference is greater than a clinically desirable target of 10% in favour of the combination therapy. To fit these specifications with a normal distribution we require a mean $\theta = 0$ and standard deviation $\tau = 0.06080$, that is $\theta \overset{d}{=} N(0, 0.003697)$.

The enthusiastic prior distribution represents the beliefs of someone who is en-thusiastic about the new combination therapy, for example a researcher who was closely involved in the development of the therapy. Suppose this researcher had a prior belief that was equivalent to specifying a prior mean equal to the desired gain in response rates, 10% in favour of the combination treatment, with the same stan-dard deviation as we just used for the sceptic. This leads to the prior distribution $\theta \overset{d}{=} N(0.1, 0.003697)$, which results in the enthusiastic prior distribution having just 5% prior probability that the true difference is less than 0.

The three prior distributions are plotted in Figure 7.2. Recall from our discussion in Section 7.7 that the non-informative prior distribution is a uniform distribution on the whole real line $(-\infty, \infty)$. Since such a distribution cannot integrate to 1, we called this distribution an improper prior distribution. The height of the improper non-informative prior distribution does not affect the shape of the posterior distribu-tion, so in Figure 7.2 we have plotted it at an arbitrary height, chosen to be $\frac{5}{3}$. This allows the non-informative prior to integrate to 1 over the interval $(-0.2, 0.4)$, which is the range of the x-axis in Figure 7.2. This facilitates a convenient comparison with the other two prior distributions.

Individually, each of these prior distributions is to some extent unrealistic, since they each represent rather extreme views. However, an advantage of looking at the conclusions implied by all of them, is that we then get a fairly wide range of results, between which most reasonable opinions could be expected to lie.

7.10.4   Bayesian analysis

As discussed in Section 7.5 for the normal model and Section 7.9 for the more gen-eral case, when we use a non-informative prior distribution with a large sample size then the posterior distribution for θ is approximately the estimated distribution of the MLE. In the present case this means that the posterior distribution is approximately

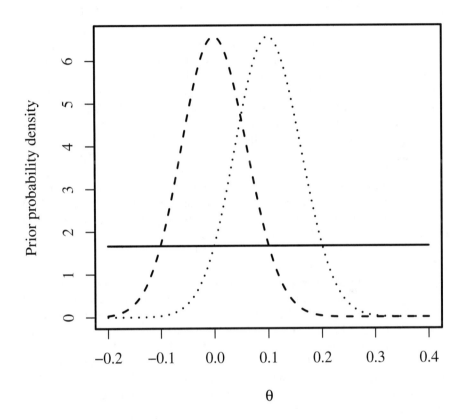

FIGURE 7.2
Prior distributions for the risk difference θ under three different prior beliefs concerning the effect of the combination treatment: non-informative (solid line), sceptical (dashed line) and enthusiastic (dotted line). The improper non-informative prior is plotted at an arbitrary height, as explained in the text.

TABLE 7.1

Posterior probability that the difference between response rates exceeds certain values, assuming three different prior distributions.

Prior distribution	$\Pr(\theta > 0.1 \mid y)$	$\Pr(\theta > 0.05 \mid y)$	$\Pr(\theta > 0 \mid y)$
non-informative	0.50	0.76	0.92
sceptical	0.11	0.44	0.82
enthusiastic	0.50	0.86	0.99

$N(0.1, 0.004942)$, using the fact that $\hat{\theta} = \hat{p}_1 - \hat{p}_0 = 0.1$ and our earlier computation of the variance 0.004942. Thus, given the concordance between the posterior distribution and the estimated distribution of the MLE, a Bayesian credible interval will be exactly the same as a conventional confidence interval, namely $(-0.03779, 0.2378)$. However, under the Bayesian approach it is the entire posterior distribution that represents our uncertainty about θ, not just the credible interval derived from the posterior distribution. The importance of this is illustrated in Figure 7.3. There it can be seen that the Bayesian posterior distribution is truly a distribution, not just an interval, so it is clear that we should put more belief in values of θ near the point estimate in the middle of the interval, relative to values nearer the ends of the interval. Furthermore, we can use the posterior distribution to make probability statements about the parameter θ. For example, we can state the probability that the true treatment difference is greater than 5%, by comparing $(0.05 - 0.1)/\sqrt{0.004942}$ with the standard normal distribution. The results of such probability calculations are displayed in Table 7.1.

Posterior distributions corresponding to the other two prior distributions can also be obtained, using the general posterior distribution for inference about a normal mean presented in Section 7.5. Under the sceptical prior distribution, the posterior distribution is normal with mean 0.04279 and standard deviation 0.04599. Similarly, for the enthusiastic prior distribution, the posterior distribution has mean 0.1 and standard deviation again 0.04599. These posterior distributions are also shown in Figure 7.3, where they can be compared with the posterior distribution corresponding to a non-informative prior distribution, and can be used for the posterior probability calculations displayed in Table 7.1.

7.10.5 Interpretation

Some statisticians would argue that the probabilities in Table 7.1 allow a more complete interpretation of the data than a frequentist analysis based on a P-value and a confidence interval. In this example the frequentist analysis, which can be thought of as equivalent to a Bayesian analysis based on a non-informative prior distribution, indicated that there was only weak evidence, if any, of a meaningful gain in response rates under the combination therapy. The Bayesian analysis allows us to ask whether this conclusion would still hold for either a sceptic or an enthusiastic supporter of the combination therapy. The posterior distributions show that the sceptic's doubts are

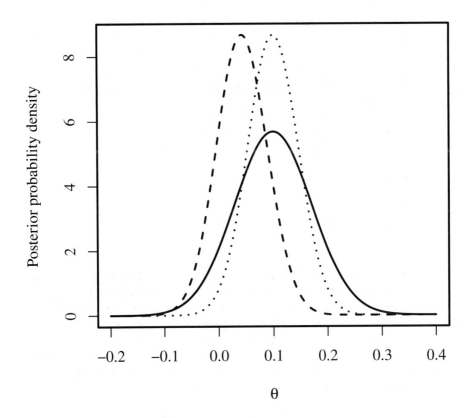

FIGURE 7.3
Posterior distributions for the risk difference θ based on the data in Table 5.2 and
the three prior distributions from Figure 7.2: non-informative (solid line), sceptical
(dashed line) and enthusiastic (dotted line).

not greatly dented by these data, since the posterior probability of a difference greater than 0.1 only increases to 11% from the prior probability of 5%. On the other hand, it is obvious that the data do not move the enthusiast's prior mean of a difference of 0.1, although they considerably strengthen the enthusiast's case that the effect is greater than 0. An impartial analyst would conclude that, although the results tend to indicate a benefit for the combination therapy, they certainly do not provide enough evidence to convince a sceptic. In this case it might be recommended that further research be conducted to accumulate more evidence.

From a qualitative point of view, the conclusions from the Bayesian analysis are not dramatically different from those reached in the extended example of Chapter 5 using a frequentist perspective. However, an important distinction is that the Bayesian approach allows the conclusions to be expressed using direct probability statements about the parameter of interest, the difference between the response rates in the two treatment groups. The Bayesian approach also allows the evidence in the data to be weighed up against a range of plausible prior opinions as to the likely benefit of the alternative therapy. Some see this as an inherent advantage of the Bayesian approach, while others believe it makes the analysis dependent on subjective assumptions. Therein lies the fundamental distinction between proponents of the Bayesian and frequentist approaches.

Exercises

1. As discussed in Example 7.1, one of the simplest example of Bayes' rule is the calculation of probabilities relating to just two alternative values of a parameter based on a single binary observation. This calculation has a standard application in clinical medicine, for obtaining the predictive value of a test result for a patient. Suppose the patient either has a disease, denoted D^+, or does not have the disease, denoted D^-. A diagnostic test can produce a positive result, denoted T^+, or a negative results, denoted T^-. Two important properties of the test are the **sensitivity** and **specificity**, denoted respectively

$$s_n = \Pr(T^+|D^+) \quad \text{and} \quad s_p = \Pr(T^-|D^-).$$

   (a) After the test has been done, what is the probability that the patient has the disease? Write down a formula for the two probabilities, corresponding to the two possible results, using Bayes' rule to express each probability in terms of the sensitivity and specificity of the test, and the pre-test probability that the patient has the disease, $\Pr(D^+)$.

   (b) Now assume that the test has sensitivity 90% and specificity 70%, and suppose that the patient has a positive test result. Create a table showing the posterior probability of disease for the following range of pre-test probabilities: $\Pr(D^+) = 0.001, 0.01, 0.1, 0.2, 0.5, 0.8$. For which of these values is a positive test result most useful? Can the test result, that is the data, be meaningfully interpreted for any individual patient without using some assumption about the pre-test probability of disease? Note that the posterior probability has a special name in the context of diagnostic testing, namely, the **positive predictive value**.

2. The beta distribution arises naturally in Bayesian estimation of proportions, as explained in the examples described in this chapter. In this exercise we consider various properties of the beta distribution in Bayesian inference, including confirming some of the results mentioned in the examples.

   (a) Confirm that the uniform distribution is a beta distribution with $\alpha = \beta = 1$. If this distribution is used as a prior distribution for estimating prevalence from data represented as an observed number of diseased individuals y and a sample size n, what are the parameters of the resulting beta posterior distribution?

   (b) Using the facts about the beta distribution given in Appendix 1, what are the mean, mode and variance of the posterior distribution?

   (c) Consider a sample of 100 children where 20 have a history of asthma. What is the posterior probability that the prevalence of asthma history in the population is greater than 15%. Find an answer under each of the following beta prior distributions. Interpret the results in each case using a plot of the prior and posterior distributions. Comment on the influence that each prior distribution has. Hence comment on the strength of the prior beliefs that each prior distribution represents.

      i. Uniform distribution $(\alpha = \beta = 1)$
      ii. $\alpha = \beta = 0.5$
      iii. $\alpha = 1, \beta = 4$
      iv. $\alpha = 1, \beta = 9$

   (d) Confirm algebraically (in general) and numerically (for the above cases), that the posterior mean for the prevalence lies between the prior mean and the observed proportion, y/n. This is a general feature of Bayesian inference, namely, that the posterior distribution is centred at a location that is a compromise between the location of the prior distribution and the information in the data. Comment on how this compromise is controlled by considering when the posterior mean will be closer to the observed proportion or to the prior mean.

3. In this exercise we consider Bayesian estimation of a normal mean with known variance, using the conjugate normal prior distribution, as discussed in Section 7.5.

   (a) Fill in the missing steps for deriving the expression for $p(\theta|y)$ in Section 7.5.1.

(b) Show that the posterior mean μ_1 in part (a) can be re-arranged into the following two alternative forms

$$\mu_1 = \mu_0 + (y - \mu_0)\frac{\tau_0^2}{\sigma^2 + \tau_0^2}$$

and

$$\mu_1 = y + (\mu_0 - y)\frac{\sigma^2}{\sigma^2 + \tau_0^2}.$$

The first expression shows the posterior mean as the prior mean plus an adjustment towards the observed y, while the second shows the posterior mean as the observed y with an adjustment towards the prior mean. Both forms indicate the essential feature of Bayesian estimation, that of the providing a compromise between the two sources of information.

4. Refer back to the fertility study discussed in the examples of Chapter 4. Recall that the data consist of n couples who take a total of y conception cycles to achieve a pregnancy. The parameter of interest is the probability θ of pregnancy within a single conception cycle. In this exercise we consider only the case of a single group, not the comparison of two groups. Notice that we using the notation θ for the probability, rather than the notation p that was used in Chapter 4, in order to avoid confusion with the Bayesian notation for prior distributions and posterior distributions.

(a) Using the likelihood function L based on the geometric distribution discussed in Example 4.1 of Chapter 4, write down the form of $p(y|\theta)$.

(b) Using part (a), show that the beta distribution is a conjugate prior for estimating the parameter θ.

(c) Find the posterior distribution for θ and compare it with the posterior distribution used in the prevalence example discussed in this chapter. Hence argue that inference for a success probability based on the number of successes and the number of trials, are the same regardless of whether the binomial or geometric sampling models are used.

(d) With reference to Example 4.2 and Figure 4.2 of Chapter 4, recall that when $y = n$ then the MLE is $\hat{\theta} = 1$. Explain how a Bayesian analysis deals with the fact that the MLE is on the boundary of the parameter space. To answer this question, experiment with some alternative prior distributions and look at the corresponding posterior distributions. This situation is a good illustration of the fact that the Bayesian analysis focuses more on producing an entire posterior distribution for the parameter, rather than a single point estimate.

5. This exercise is based on the extended example described in Section 7.10, which used the data from Table 5.2 of Chapter 5. Now suppose that the study described is continued until the sample size has doubled, with the resulting data given below.

	Mono-therapy	Combination therapy	Total
Response	$x_0 = 90$	$x_1 = 114$	204
No response	108	88	196
Total	$n_0 = 198$	$n_1 = 202$	$n = 400$

(a) Work out the three posterior distributions for the difference in response rates, as in Section 7.10, based on the new data. Obtain the posterior probability of the difference being greater than 0, 0.05 and 0.1, as in Table 7.1. How do the interpretations change, from the perspective of the sceptic and the enthusiast?

(b) Consider now a "realistic" prior distribution, which is normal in shape, but allows for a 20% probability that the difference is negative (favouring the control mono-therapy group) and 20% probability that it is greater than 0.1. Determine the appropriate parameters for this normal distribution, and obtain the corresponding posterior distribution and posterior probabilities. How different are the conclusions from this fourth distribution to those obtained under each of the previous three prior distributions?

6. In Section 4.8.2 of Chapter 4 we discussed a single sample of n patients for the purpose of estimating the incidence rate of stroke, $\theta > 0$. The data consist of y stroke events observed in a total of F person-years of follow-up. We will assume that at least one stroke was observed in the sample, so $y \geq 1$.

(a) Assuming that y is an observation from a Poisson distributed random variable, write down the form of the likelihood, $p(y|\theta)$, for this model.

(b) Consider the following prior distribution

$$p(\theta) \propto \theta^{\alpha-1} \exp(-\beta\theta) \qquad \text{for } \theta > 0$$

which has two parameters $\alpha > 0$ and $\beta > 0$. This is called the gamma distribution, Gamma(α, β), which is reviewed in Appendix 1. Show that the gamma prior distribution is the conjugate prior distribution for this model.

(c) Find the posterior distribution $p(\theta|y)$ and express it as a gamma distribution.

(d) Using properties of the gamma distribution, derive the maximum posterior estimate of the stroke incidence rate, and the mean of the posterior distribution for the stroke incidence rate. Compare and comment on these two point estimates.

(e) What is the MLE of the stroke incidence rate? What prior distribution would make the maximum posterior estimate be equivalent to the MLE of the stroke incidence rate?

8

Further inference topics

In this final chapter we present a range of topics that go beyond our main focus of likelihood-based inference for parametric models with large samples. The intention is not to provide a complete presentation of these topics but rather to give a brief introduction to approaches that can be used without making parametric or large sample assumptions. We begin with exact methods that make use of the actual sampling distribution in small samples rather than normal or χ^2 approximations for large samples. We then describe non-parametric methods that require no assumptions, or at least very few assumptions, about the probability distribution that generated our sample. We also discuss an important class of computer-intensive methods called resampling methods, particularly bootstrapping. While the presentation is necessarily cursory, our discussion provides a taste of the breadth of additional inference topics required by practising biostatisticians. The methods are illustrated by reconsidering a number of our earlier examples from these alternative perspectives.

8.1 Exact methods

In our discussions of estimation and hypothesis testing in previous chapters we made use of the sampling distributions of estimators and test statistics to understand the properties of the associated estimation and testing procedures. The primary tool for determining these sampling distributions was the asymptotic distribution of the MLE, which provides a general unified approach to inference in large samples using an approximate normal or χ^2-distribution. While this approach is useful in that it applies to a broad variety of parametric models, it has the disadvantage of relying on an approximation that requires the sample to be "large". In this section we briefly introduce the concept of exact statistical inference, which is an approach that is applicable for any sample size, no matter how small.

Exact methods make use of the actual, or exact, sampling distribution for constructing estimation and testing procedures. A simple example of the distinction between an exact sampling distribution and one based on a normal approximation has already been discussed, in Example 1.7 of Chapter 1. In that example we discussed the sampling distribution of the prevalence estimator P, which is the proportion of individuals infected in a random sample of n individuals from a population of interest. Using the usual binomial model for the number infected in the sample, the large sample normal approximation for the sampling distribution was given as

$$P \overset{d}{\approx} \mathrm{N}\left(\theta, \frac{\theta(1-\theta)}{n}\right)$$

whereas the exact distribution was defined in terms of the discrete probability function

$$f_P(p; \theta) = \Pr(P = p) = \frac{n!}{(n-pn)!(pn)!}\theta^{pn}(1-\theta)^{n-pn} \qquad p = 0, \frac{1}{n}, \frac{2}{n}, \ldots, 1.$$

Notice that the large sample approximation involves using a continuous distribution to approximate a discrete distribution. For large n this works well but for small n the exact sampling distribution is highly discrete and we can expect substantive differences between the approximate and exact distributions. These differences may even include non-zero probability for impossible values of P that are outside the range $[0,1]$ when using the normal approximation. This is illustrated for a specific small sample context in Figure 8.1, where we have plotted the exact probability function for the random variable P, along with its normal approximation. We will study these differences further in the exercises.

Since the exact and approximate sampling distributions may differ in small samples, the large sample approximation may lead to invalid inference if the sample is small enough. It is therefore of interest to consider inference procedures based on the exact distribution, which will remain valid even if the sample is small. In fact, we have already seen an example of an inference method that uses an exact distribution in preference to a large sample approximation, namely, the ubiquitous t-test. The t-test, in its various one-sample and two-sample forms, uses an exact sampling distribution that accommodates the extra variability introduced by having to estimate the population variance in the test statistic, whereas the corresponding large sample normal approximation ignores this variability. While this is an important example of an exact method, in practice, most of the common exact methods are designed to deal with discrete contexts in which the continuous large sample approximation is a poor approximation to a highly discrete small sample sampling distribution. A comprehensive discussion of these exact methods is beyond our scope, but the above binomial model provides an exemplar which will be used here to illustrate the basic ideas.

We will start by considering exact inference for the binomial prevalence model, which will also obviously include inference for any other one-sample binomial context. For a population prevalence θ and a specific null value θ_0, consider a one-sided test of the hypotheses

$$\mathrm{H}_0 : \theta = \theta_0 \qquad \text{versus} \qquad \mathrm{H}_1 : \theta < \theta_0.$$

Clearly, we will want to reject the null hypothesis in favour of the alternative hypothesis if the observed prevalence is sufficiently low. Thus, a one-sided test at significance level α will involve rejecting H_0 if the observed prevalence p satisfies $p \leq c(\alpha; \theta_0)$, where $c(\alpha; \theta_0)$ is an appropriate critical value that depends on both the significance

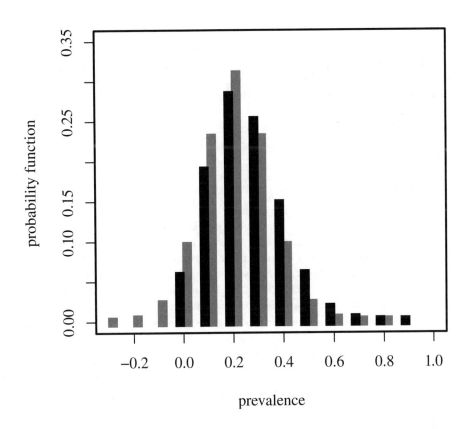

FIGURE 8.1
Comparison of the exact (dark) and approximate (light) sampling distributions for the prevalence P in a sample of $n = 10$ individuals with population prevalence $\theta = 0.2$

level α and the null parameter value θ_0. If we were using the large sample normal approximation, then this critical value would be straightforwardly obtained as

$$c(\alpha; \theta_0) = \theta_0 + z_\alpha \sqrt{\frac{\theta_0(1 - \theta_0)}{n}}.$$

This definition ensures that the probability of rejecting H_0 when H_0 is true is equal to the desired significance level

$$\Pr\left(P \leq c(\alpha; \theta_0) \mid \theta = \theta_0\right) = \Phi\left(\frac{c(\alpha; \theta_0) - \theta_0}{\sqrt{\theta_0(1 - \theta_0)/n}}\right) = \alpha$$

where Φ is the standard normal cumulative distribution function.

The same approach could in principle be used to obtain an exact test, by using the exact sampling distribution instead of its large sample normal approximation. This requires us to use the exact probability function specified earlier in this section, $f_P(p; \theta)$, and its corresponding cumulative distribution function, $F_P(p; \theta)$. We could then define the critical value similarly to the above large sample definition, such that the probability of rejecting H_0 when H_0 is true is equal to the desired significance level

$$\Pr\left(P \leq c(\alpha; \theta_0) \mid \theta = \theta_0\right) = F_P\left(c(\alpha; \theta_0)\right) = \sum_{x \leq c(\alpha;\theta_0)} f_P(x; \theta_0) = \alpha.$$

However, although this would be the ideal way to define the critical value, in practice the discreteness of the exact sampling distribution introduces a problem that was not present when we used the continuous normal approximation. In particular, because of the discreteness of the distribution it may not be possible to find a $c(\alpha; \theta_0)$ such that the significance level is precisely equal to α. For this reason we have to modify the approach taken in the continuous case, and choose $c(\alpha; \theta_0)$ as large as possible such that the significance level of the test is as close as possible to α without exceeding α. That is,

$$c(\alpha; \theta_0) = \max\left\{y : \sum_{x \leq y} f_P(x; \theta_0) \leq \alpha\right\}.$$

We return below to the importance of accommodating the discreteness of the sampling distribution in this and many other exact inference contexts.

The above basic approach can be modified in various ways. For example, a one-sided exact test in the opposite direction is obtained by simply reversing the direction of the critical value definition, so that H_0 is rejected if $p \geq d(\alpha; \theta_0)$ where

$$d(\alpha; \theta_0) = \min\left\{y : \sum_{x \geq y} f_P(x; \theta_0) \leq \alpha\right\}.$$

A two-sided exact test is then obtained by using the intersection of the two one-sided tests, each with significance level $\alpha/2$. That is, we reject H_0 if

$$p \leq c\left(\frac{\alpha}{2}; \theta_0\right) \qquad \text{or} \qquad p \geq d\left(\frac{\alpha}{2}; \theta_0\right).$$

Furthermore, a confidence interval can be obtained by using the test-based confidence interval approach discussed in Section 6.10 of Chapter 6. In particular, a confidence interval with a confidence level of at least $100(1 - \alpha)\%$ consists of the range of θ_0 values such that the two-sided exact test would not reject the null hypothesis. Although the tests and confidence interval are fairly straightforward to define, notice that the computations themselves are not straightforward because c and d are only defined implicitly as the solution of somewhat complicated equations. Nonetheless, standard statistical software packages are able to undertake these computations, as illustrated in Example 8.1 below.

Before considering an example, we note that the need to take account of the discreteness of the sampling distribution highlights an important complication that arises with many exact methods. When the sampling distribution is discrete, then exact methods can be considered exact in the sense that they use the actual sampling distribution, but they may be unable to provide an exact significance level or confidence level due to the discreteness of the underlying sampling distribution. Thus, for example, it may not be possible to provide an exact 95% confidence interval or an exact hypothesis test at the 5% significance level. In such cases it is necessary to err on the side of conservatism, so exact methods will be conservative in the sense that they lead to a higher confidence level, or lower significance level, than is desired. Importantly though, this does not mean that the exact methods produce invalid results, it simply reflects a restriction on the nature of the exact analysis that can be conducted. For example, it may only be possible to construct a 96.1% confidence interval rather than the desired 95% confidence interval, but we can rest assured that the 96.1% confidence is valid in the sense that its coverage probability will be 0.961. This conservatism tends to be more of an issue in highly discrete settings, such as would occur with very small sizes, and tends to diminish as the sample size increases.

Example 8.1 In Example 2.5, we discussed confidence intervals for the population prevalence using the large sample normal approximation to the binomial distribution. In particular, in Table 2.1 we presented the confidence intervals that would arise for different sample sizes and different values of the observed prevalence p. Table 8.1 expands on Table 2.1 by presenting the exact confidence intervals, as well as an additional prevalence value $p = 0.01$. It can be seen from Table 8.1 that for small samples with low prevalence the normal approximation does not work well, in the sense that it leads to confidence intervals that do not provide a good approximation to the exact confidence intervals. Indeed, in this case it may even lead to ranges that include impossible negative values for the population prevalence. However, it can also be seen that for other combinations of sample size and prevalence, the approximation is quite good. This is particularly true when our rule of thumb $n \geq 20/p$ is satisfied. Note that the smallest sample size considered in Table 8.1 is $n = 100$, which would often not be considered particularly small. However, when this sample size is combined with a very low prevalence value then it is seen to be insufficient to produce a good approximation. Smaller samples, particularly when combined with low prevalence values, would lead the approximation to perform even worse.

TABLE 8.1

95% confidence intervals for the population prevalence (%) based on various scenarios for the observed sample prevalence (p) and the sample size (n), using both exact and approximate methods

p	Approximate		Exact	
	$n = 100$	$n = 1000$	$n = 100$	$n = 1000$
0.01	$-1.0 - 3.0$	$0.4 - 1.6$	$0.0 - 5.5$	$0.5 - 1.8$
0.05	$0.7 - 9.3$	$3.6 - 6.4$	$1.6 - 11.3$	$3.7 - 6.5$
0.10	$4.1 - 15.9$	$8.1 - 11.9$	$4.9 - 17.6$	$8.2 - 12.0$
0.25	$16.5 - 33.5$	$22.3 - 27.7$	$16.9 - 34.7$	$22.3 - 27.8$
0.50	$40.2 - 59.8$	$46.9 - 53.1$	$39.8 - 60.2$	$46.9 - 53.2$

The previous discussion illustrates exact inference for one-sample binomial models. Exact inference methods are also available for two-sample binomial models, where the goal is to test the equality of two probabilities. An example of approximate large sample inference for this context was discussed at some length in the extended example of Chapter 5, and the same example could be handled using an exact inference approach. In particular, one of the primary exact inference tools for two-sample binomial models is an hypothesis testing method referred to as **Fisher's exact test**, named after the statistician R.A. Fisher. For understanding Fisher's exact test it is helpful to view the data in the form of a 2×2 table with row totals and column totals, as depicted in Table 5.2 of the Chapter 5 extended example. The basis of Fisher's exact test is to consider the probability, under the null hypothesis of equality of the binomial probabilities, of each possible 2×2 configuration that could give rise to the same row and column totals as the observed data. If the observed 2×2 configuration is extreme relative to the distribution of possible configurations, then this provides a basis on which to reject the null hypothesis of equality of the two binomial proportions. It turns out that the probability of any particular 2×2 configuration can be specified using the hypergeometric distribution, which is described in Appendix 1. In particular, using the notation in Table 5.2, the probability associated with any particular 2×2 table is given by the hypergeometric probability

$$\frac{\binom{x_0+x_1}{x_0}\binom{n-x_0-x_1}{n_0-x_0}}{\binom{n}{n_0}} = \frac{(x_0+x_1)!(n-x_0-x_1)!n_0!n_1!}{x_0!x_1!(n_0-x_0)!(n_1-x_1)!n!}.$$

This amounts to viewing x_0 as the number of individuals who have a particular trait, in a random sample of size n_0 individuals from a population of size n individuals, $x_0 + x_1$ of whom have the particular trait. Thus, in addition to viewing the sample size n as a fixed constant, we are effectively also viewing the column total n_0 and the row total $x_0 + x_1$ as fixed constants. We return to this assumption later in the section.

With the hypergeometric probability assigned to any possible 2×2 configuration, the P-value for Fisher's exact test is obtained by determining this probability for all possible 2×2 configurations and then summing up the probabilities that are less than or equal to the probability associated with the observed 2×2 table. In very small samples there are very few possible 2×2 configurations so it is possible to do these calculations by hand, and we will illustrate this process in the exercises. For larger samples, the calculations quickly become unwieldy and it is necessary to make use of one of the many standard statistical analysis software packages that implement Fisher's exact test.

Example 8.2 For the extended example of Chapter 5, we can apply Fisher's exact test to the 2×2 table of response and no response data presented in Table 5.2. For example, under the null hypothesis of equality of the response rates, the probability of observing the 2×2 configuration displayed in Table 5.2, from among all possible configurations with the same row and column totals, is the hypergeometric probability

$$\frac{\binom{47+57}{47}\binom{200-47-57}{100-47}}{\binom{200}{100}} = 0.042.$$

In total there are 101 possible 2×2 configurations with the same row and column totals, and the P-value for Fisher's exact test is calculated by adding up all of the associated hypergeometric probabilities that are at least as extreme as the observed sample, that is, less than or equal to 0.042. This produces a P-value of 0.20, which can be compared to the P-value computed using the large sample approximation in Chapter 5, which was 0.16. The two P-values in this case are not particularly different, and would produce the same conclusion when used for an hypothesis test, namely, that there is no evidence to reject the null hypothesis. This is perhaps not too surprising for this particular example, because the overall sample size of $n = 200$ is large enough for the normal distribution to be a good approximation. With smaller samples, however, the exact and approximate methods may show more substantial differences.

Observe that in implementing Fisher's exact test in Example 8.2 we only considered whether the observed sample was extreme relative to 2×2 configurations that have the same row and column totals as the observed sample in Table 5.2. Why did we only consider configurations having these particular row and column totals? The reason is that, even if the row and column totals are not really fixed, they are statistics that have distributions that do not depend on the parameter of interest, the difference in response rates. Such a statistic is called an **ancillary statistic** and is essentially the opposite of a sufficient statistic. Whereas a sufficient statistic captures all of the available information about the parameter, an ancillary statistic provides no information about the parameter. Our inferences can therefore be carried out after conditioning on the value of the ancillary statistic, or in other words treating it as if it were a fixed constant like the sample size n. The topic of ancillary statistics and conditional inference is an important advanced topic in the theory of statistical inference and is taken up in more detail by some of the texts on mathematical statistics described in Appendix 3.

In this section we have introduced the basic concept of using the exact sampling distribution rather than the large sample normal approximation, in order to produce methods that are valid for small as well as large sample sizes. While this has some obvious advantages in small samples, a disadvantage is that there is no longer a unified approach to determining an appropriate sampling distribution. This means that exact methods tend to require theoretical justifications that are specific to the context and generally require greater complexity compared to the simplicity of the normal approximation, both in terms of theoretical development and computational resources. For this reason, exact methods tend to be used primarily for small samples where their advantages are worth the complexity. An obvious practical issue for the use of exact methods is how to define a small sample. There is no single answer to this question, and guidelines are often developed in specific contexts. For example, in Section 2.7 we mentioned a rule of thumb for using the normal approximation to the binomial distribution, which required a sample size of $n \geq 20/p$. As illustrated in Example 8.1 this rule often works well in practice. Generally these types of guidelines are developed based on theoretical or simulation studies that investigate how well the normal distribution approximates the exact sampling distribution in specific contexts.

8.2   Non-parametric methods

The methods that we discussed in other chapters were based on parametric statistical models. We introduced parametric models in Section 2.2, where we described them as models that assume the distribution takes a specific form which is fully known except for a small number of fixed constants called parameters. We have discussed various parametric models in this book, based on distributions such as the normal or binomial distributions, and we have discussed various methods for estimating and testing hypotheses about the unknown parameters in these distributions.

Assuming a known parametric form is clearly an important assumption that may not always be true. Making the wrong parametric assumption can invalidate our inferences, so when we do not know the sampling distribution it is natural to seek methods that do not require an assumption about this distribution. **Non-parametric methods** are methods that allow us to undertake statistical inference without making an assumption that the sample has been taken from a particular distribution, such as the normal distribution. These methods are also sometimes called **distribution-free methods**, because they are free of the assumption that the distribution of the sample is known.

One of the most basic non-parametric methods is an approach for estimating the cumulative distribution function of the probability distribution that the sample was taken from. Consider the sample values $y_1, \ldots, y_n$ which are the observed values of independent and identically distributed random variables $Y_1, \ldots, Y_n$ having an unknown probability distribution with cumulative distribution function $F(y) = \Pr(Y_i \leq y)$. We have already seen methods of estimation that allow us to estimate the cumulative distribution function, and hence other aspects of the probability distribution, when using a parametric model. For example, if we assume a parametric model based on the $N(\mu, \sigma^2)$ distribution, then plugging in the sample mean $\bar{y}$ and sample variance s_{n-1}^2 as estimates of μ and σ^2, respectively, will yield an estimate of $F(y)$ using the cumulative distribution function from the normal $N(\bar{y}, s_{n-1}^2)$ distribution. In contrast, the **empirical distribution function** $\hat{F}_n(y)$ is an estimate of $F(y)$ that makes no assumption about the underlying distribution of the sample. The empirical cumulative distribution function is defined as

$$\hat{F}_n(y) = \frac{\sum_{i=1}^{n} 1\{y_i \leq y\}}{n} \qquad y \in (-\infty, \infty)$$

where $1\{\cdot\}$ is an indicator function that takes the value 1 if the condition inside the brackets is true and 0 otherwise. Thus, the numerator of this definition is the number of observations that have values less than or equal to y, and $\hat{F}_n(y)$ is therefore simply the proportion of the sample that is less than or equal to y.

Notice that the empirical distribution function will always be constant in between the observed sample values and that it takes a jump upwards at each sample value. The size of the jump at a particular sample value will depend on the sample size n and the number of observations that have that sample value. If all observations in the sample have different values then the size of each jump will be $\frac{1}{n}$, whereas the jump may be larger if multiple observations have the same value. Because of the appearance of the empirical distribution function when plotted, it is often referred to as a **step-function**, as illustrated in Figure 8.2 of the following example.

Example 8.3 In the extended example discussed in Section 2.10 of Chapter 2, we considered a sample of cholesterol levels taken on $n = 100$ individuals. We used the histogram plotted in Figure 2.2 as an indication that the normal distribution would provide an appropriate parametric model for the sample. Such an assessment can also be conducted using the empirical distribution function. The empirical distribution function from this sample is plotted in Figure 8.2. This plot illustrates the form of the step-function, which consists of a sequence of constant segments with jumps corresponding to the observed cholesterol levels in the sample. The sample mean and variance for this sample are $\bar{y} = 5.26$ and $s_{n-1}^2 = 0.48$. Also plotted in Figure 8.2 is the cumulative distribution function from the $N(5.26, 0.48)$ distribution. Since the empirical distribution function is free to follow whatever shape the sample observations require, the fact that the estimated normal distribution closely follows the empirical distribution function provides support for the use of a parametric model based on the normal distribution. In other samples it may be that the estimated normal distribution does not follow the empirical distribution very closely, which would suggest that a parametric model based on the normal distribution may provide misleading inferences. This highlights an important use of non-parametric methods, namely, that they can provide guidance on an appropriate parametric model for the sample.

In the exercises of Chapter 5 we considered an alternative to the one-sample t-

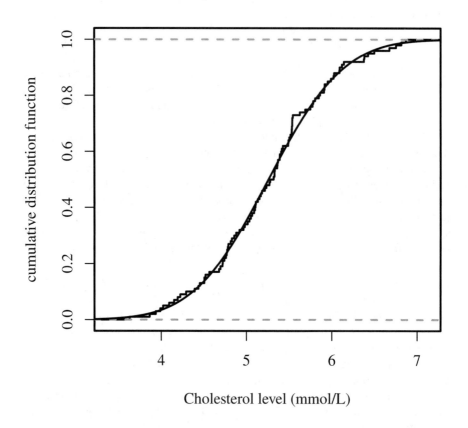

FIGURE 8.2
Empirical distribution function for the sample of cholesterol levels plotted in Figure
2.2. Also plotted is the cumulative distribution function from the estimated parametric model based on the normal distribution

test for testing whether a population mean is equal to zero using a single sample. This test was referred to as the **Wilcoxon signed-rank test**, which is named after Frank Wilcoxon, the statistician that first suggested the test. Although we studied the properties of the test using simulation, we did not discuss the specifics of how the test is carried out. In fact, the Wilcoxon signed-rank test is a prime example of a non-parametric test, particularly because it illustrates the use of sample ranks to conduct inferences, which is a common approach in non-parametric methods.

The Wilcoxon signed-rank test allows us to test whether the population mean θ is zero, under the assumption that the distribution of the sample is symmetric. Thus, although we will not need to make an assumption about the specific form of the distribution, we do make an assumption that it is symmetric. Also note that since we are assuming that the distribution is symmetric, θ can also be interpreted as the median. The hypotheses to be tested are

$$H_0 : \theta = 0 \quad \text{versus} \quad H_1 : \theta \neq 0.$$

The null hypothesis $\theta = 0$ may seem restrictive, however, any other simple null hypothesis $\theta = \theta_0$ can also be used, simply by applying the test to the shifted observations $y_1 - \theta_0, \ldots, y_n - \theta_0$.

With these assumptions, the Wilcoxon signed-rank test uses just the signs and the ranks of the observations in the sample. The sign of observation i denotes whether the observation is positive or negative, taking the value 1 or -1 respectively,

$$\text{sign}(y_i) = \begin{cases} 1 & \text{if } y_i > 0 \\ 0 & \text{if } y_i = 0 \\ -1 & \text{if } y_i < 0. \end{cases}$$

The rank of an observation denotes the position in the sample that the observation takes when the sample is ranked from smallest to largest. Thus, the smallest observation has rank 1 and the largest observation has rank n. Where two or more observations have identical values, each observation is assigned the average of the ranks that the observations cover. The Wilcoxon signed-rank test actually uses the ranks of the absolute values of the sample, $\text{rank}(|y_i|)$. If the null hypothesis is true and the sample comes from a symmetric distribution, then we would expect $\text{sign}(y_i)\text{rank}(|y_i|)$ to be distributed symmetrically around 0. This suggests the following statistic for testing the null hypothesis

$$t_{SR} = \sum_{i=1}^{n} \text{sign}(y_i)\text{rank}(|y_i|).$$

Clearly t_{SR} will tend to be close to 0 if the null hypothesis is true, and if t_{SR} departs too far from 0 in either direction then this would reflect a departure from the null hypothesis. In fact, t_{SR} is the observed value of a random variable T_{SR} that has an exact distribution that can be enumerated for smaller samples, and an approximate normal distribution in larger samples. Thus, these distributions can be used to specify the rejection rule for testing the null hypothesis. For the exact distribution, the critical value for the hypothesis test can be obtained in many standard software packages, while for the approximate normal distribution the test with significance level α is

Wilcoxon signed-rank test :   reject H_0 if $|t_{SR}| \geq z_{1-\alpha/2}\sqrt{\dfrac{n(n+1)(2n+1)}{6}}$

where z_x is the x-percentile of the standard normal distribution. This critical value follows from the following approximate normal distribution under the null hypothesis,

$$T_{SR} \overset{d}{\approx} N\left(0, \frac{n(n+1)(2n+1)}{6}\right).$$

This distribution can also be used in an obvious way for calculating P-values and for obtaining an analogous one-sided test.

The above testing procedure uses only the signs and the ranks of the sample values, and not the actual sample values. This means that not all information in the sample is being used. The trade-off for using only part of the information in the sample is that we can avoid making a specific parametric assumption about the form of the distribution, albeit still requiring a much weaker assumption that the distribution is symmetric. Even this assumption can be dispensed with if we are prepared to further reduce the amount of information that is used from the sample. For example, if we just use the signs of the observations, and interpret θ as the median of the distribution, then the number of positive signs has a $Bin(n, 0.5)$ distribution under the null hypothesis. This distribution can then be used to construct a test of the null hypothesis, which is referred to as the **sign test**. The sign test avoids the assumption of symmetry, but this comes at an even greater cost in terms of lost information. We will study the sign test further in the exercises, but for now we consider an example based on the Wilcoxon signed-rank test.

Example 8.4 In the exercises of Chapter 5 we considered a study in which HIV infected individuals were given six months of antiviral therapy and the reduction in their HIV viral load was measured. Table 8.2 lists a sample $n = 25$ viral load reduction measurements in which the sample mean reduction is $\bar{y} = 0.251$ and sample variance is $s_{n-1}^2 = 0.784$. Also provided are various quantities required to carry out the Wilcoxon signed-rank test, which in this case would test the null hypothesis that the mean or median reduction is zero. The observed value of the test statistic is $t_{SR} = 161$, which is the sum of the right hand column of Table 8.2. Since $n = 25$, the variance of the normal distribution under the null hypothesis is

$$\frac{n(n+1)(2n+1)}{6} = \frac{25 \times 26 \times 51}{6} = 5525$$

which yields a critical value of $1.96 \times \sqrt{5525} = 145.69$ for the two-sided test at a significance level of $\alpha = 0.05$. This test would therefore reject the null hypothesis, since $|t_{SR}|$ exceeds the critical value, and the two-sided P-value can be calculated using the standard normal cumulative distribution function Φ,

$$2P = 1 - \Phi\left(\frac{161}{\sqrt{5525}}\right)$$

which yields $P = 0.0303$. The P-value from the exact sampling distribution for the test statistic under the null hypothesis can be obtained from standard software and yields $P = 0.0296$, which is virtually identical to the P-value based on the normal approximation. Furthermore, the sample mean and variance can be used to carry out a one-sample t-test on the data, which leads to a rather different P-value of 0.168. Since the parametric and non-parametric methods yield different conclusions, it is of interest to investigate whether the parametric assumption of normality of the viral load reductions is appropriate for this sample. Figure 8.3 displays the empirical distribution function together with the corresponding normal cumulative distribution function based on the sample mean and variance. It can be seen that the non-parametric estimate displays considerable departure from normality. It is therefore not surprising that the two tests give different results, and our investigations of the power of the two tests in the Chapter 5 exercises would suggest that the non-parametric approach is preferred in this context. Note that whereas Example 8.3 illustrated the use of the non-parametric empirical distribution function to guide the choice of an appropriate parametric model, this example has illustrated its use in identifying the inappropriateness of a particular parametric model.

Non-parametric hypothesis tests, such as those discussed above, have an obvious advantage over parametric hypothesis tests in that they do not require us to make assumptions that may turn out to be wrong and invalidate our inferences. Furthermore, non-parametric testing procedures can be extended to allow estimation and confidence interval construction for key aspects of the population. This process is analogous to the test-based confidence intervals that were discussed for parametric methods in Chapter 6 and provide a similar insensitivity to the strong assumptions inherent in parametric methods.

Nonetheless, the advantages of non-parametric methods do come at a cost. In particular, when a valid parametric model is available then non-parametric methods will typically be less informative than parametric methods, in the sense that they will have lower efficiency and power for estimation and hypothesis testing. A desirable non-parametric method is therefore one that admits only a very small loss of information. In the exercises of Chapter 5 we considered this issue for the Wilcoxon signed-rank test, in order to assess how it performs relative to its parametric competitor, the one-sample t-test. Those results showed that the Wilcoxon signed-rank test is an example of a desirable non-parametric method, in that it is able to provide the advantages of being distribution-free without losing much information.

In many contexts, the ranks of the sample contain almost as much information as the sample values themselves. Like the Wilcoxon signed-rank test, many other common non-parametric methods are based on the sample ranks and perform well compared to their parametric counterparts. In particular, a rank-based two-sample version of the Wilcoxon signed-rank test can be developed for testing the equality of two population medians, which can be considered a non-parametric counterpart to the two-sample t-test. This test is referred to as the **Wilcoxon rank-sum test**, or sometimes as the **Wilcoxon-Mann-Whitney test**. Given two independent samples, $x_1, \ldots, x_m$ and $y_1, \ldots, y_n$, from two populations having medians θ_1 and θ_2, the test is

TABLE 8.2
Sample of 25 reductions in HIV viral load during six months of
antiviral therapy together with various quantities required to
carry out the Wilcoxon signed-rank test

y_i	$\text{sign}(y_i)$	$|y_i|$	$\text{rank}(|y_i|)$	$\text{sign}(y_i) \times \text{rank}(|y_i|)$
−1.738	−1	1.738	24	−24
−0.784	−1	0.784	21	−21
−0.495	−1	0.495	19	−19
−0.334	−1	0.334	14	−14
−0.057	−1	0.057	4	−4
0.014	1	0.014	1	1
0.041	1	0.041	2	2
0.047	1	0.047	3	3
0.132	1	0.132	5	5
0.147	1	0.147	6	6
0.165	1	0.165	7	7
0.166	1	0.166	8	8
0.182	1	0.182	9	9
0.197	1	0.197	10	10
0.211	1	0.211	11	11
0.226	1	0.226	12	12
0.243	1	0.243	13	13
0.384	1	0.384	15	15
0.394	1	0.394	16	16
0.408	1	0.408	17	17
0.428	1	0.428	18	18
0.592	1	0.592	20	20
0.840	1	0.840	22	22
1.329	1	1.329	23	23
3.549	1	3.549	25	25

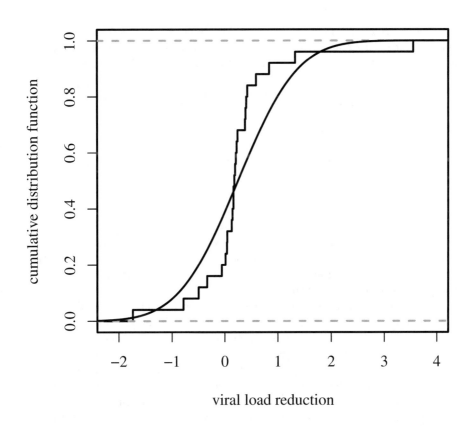

FIGURE 8.3
Empirical distribution function for the sample of viral load reductions provided in
Table 8.2. Also plotted is the cumulative distribution function from the estimated
parametric model based on the normal distribution

based on the ranks of either one of the samples within the combined sample of $n+m$ observations. That is, if we let $\text{rank}(x_i)$ be the rank of the observation x_i within the combined sample, then the test is based on the statistic

$$t_{RS} = \sum_{i=1}^{m} \text{rank}(x_i)$$

and the hypotheses to be tested are

$$H_0 : \theta_1 = \theta_2 \quad \text{versus} \quad H_1 : \theta_1 \neq \theta_2.$$

Like t_{SR}, t_{RS} is the observed value of a random variable T_{RS} that has an exact distribution that can be enumerated for smaller samples, and has an approximate normal distribution in larger samples. The approximate normal distribution under the null hypothesis is

$$T_{RS} \overset{d}{\approx} N\left(\frac{m(n+m+1)}{2}, \frac{nm(n+m+1)}{12}\right).$$

This leads to a test with significance level α

Wilcoxon rank-sum test :   reject H_0 if $\left| t_{RS} - \dfrac{m(n+m+1)}{2} \right| \geq z_{1-\alpha/2} S_{nm}$

where

$$S_{nm} = \sqrt{\frac{nm(n+m+1)}{12}}.$$

An equivalent test is based on the rank sums from the y_i observations, in which case the roles of n and m are reversed in the above description. As for the Wilcoxon signed-rank test, P-values and an analogous one-sided test can also be obtained using the approximate normal distribution.

The approach of using the ranks of the sample, rather than the values themselves, extends further to a wide class of non-parametric methods for more complex inference contexts. For example, **rank regression** is a technique that can be used as a non-parametric alternative to linear regression based on the assumption of a normally distributed sample, as was introduced in Section 4.7.1. In general, rank-based non-parametric methods can be considered to be part of a wider class of **robust methods**, which are statistical inference methods that provide valid inferences even when the underlying distribution is unknown or has been assumed to take the wrong form. The basic philosophy of all these methods is that flexibility and insensitivity to parametric assumptions can be achieved by tolerating a small cost in terms of efficiency, power and computational complexity.

8.3   Bootstrapping

There is a large class of inference procedures based on the notion of **resampling**, which means using the observed sample to generate new samples that can be used to obtain information about the properties of a particular inference procedure. As we shall see, these new samples can be generated from the original sample in a variety of ways, depending on the context. One of the most important resampling methods is **bootstrapping**, which derives its name from the idea that using the sample itself to reveal the properties of an inference procedure is akin to pulling oneself up by the bootstraps. We will discuss some of the concepts behind bootstrapping in this section, and then briefly touch on some of the other resampling methods in the next section.

Bootstrapping is essentially a method to estimate the sampling distribution of an estimator, and hence to obtain information about the properties of the estimator. One of the most important uses of bootstrapping is to quantify the variability of the estimator's sampling distribution, which can then be used for standard error and confidence interval estimation. Bootstrapping can therefore be seen as an alternative approach to parametric methods discussed elsewhere in this book, particularly those based on the information matrix associated with an MLE. Bootstrapping can often produce more accurate standard errors and confidence intervals than those based on the information matrix, without the need to make parametric assumptions but usually requiring greater computational complexity.

Before discussing how we can use resampling to implement bootstrapping, we begin with a discussion of the underlying motivation behind bootstrapping. In fact, the fundamental motivation for bootstrapping has nothing to do with resampling, although in practice it is almost always implemented using resampling. Bootstrapping involves viewing a parameter, such as the population mean or variance, as a function of the population cumulative distribution function. Consider an independent random sample $y_1, \ldots, y_n$, which are the observed values of random variables $Y_1, \ldots, Y_n$ having either a discrete or continuous distribution with cumulative distribution function F. Then any parameter of interest related to this distribution can be considered to be a function of F. For example, in Chapter 1 we wrote down a unified form for the expectation of a random variable which specifies the population mean $\mu = \mathrm{E}(Y_i)$ as a function of F

$$\mu = M(F) = \int y \, dF(y) = \begin{cases} \sum_y y f(y) & \text{for a discrete distribution} \\ \int y f(y) \, dy & \text{for a continuous distribution.} \end{cases}$$

That is, $M(F)$ is equivalent to either of the familiar summation or integral forms of the mean, depending on whether F specifies a discrete or continuous distribution, with f being either the probability function or probability density function, respectively. Likewise, the population variance $\sigma^2 = \mathrm{E}(Y_i^2) - \mathrm{E}(Y_i)^2$ is a function of F,

$$\sigma^2 = V(F) = \int y^2 \, dF(y) - \left(\int y \, dF(y) \right)^2.$$

More generally, any parameter θ can be considered a function of the function F, that is,

$$\theta = T(F).$$

As T is a function defined on the space of cumulative distribution functions, it is technically referred to as a **statistical functional**, although this mathematical terminology is peripheral to our discussion here.

Viewing θ as a function of the population cumulative distribution function F, the basic idea behind bootstrapping is to replace F by its non-parametric sample estimate, the empirical distribution function $\hat{F}_n(y)$, which was discussed in Section 8.2. This leads to a bootstrap estimate

$$\hat{\theta} = T\left(\hat{F}_n\right)$$

and the sampling distribution from which $\hat{F}_n$ was drawn then implies a sampling distribution corresponding to $\hat{\theta}$. For example, using the above specification of the mean μ, the corresponding estimate is

$$\hat{\mu} = M\left(\hat{F}_n\right) = \int y\, d\hat{F}_n(y) = \sum_{i=1}^{n} y_i\left(\frac{1}{n}\right) = \bar{y}$$

and likewise $\hat{\sigma}^2 = V\left(\hat{F}_n\right) = s_n^2$.

In practice, it is usually very complex to use the theoretical sampling distribution corresponding to $\hat{F}_n$ to lead to a theoretical sampling distribution corresponding to $T(\hat{F}_n)$. Instead, the sampling distribution corresponding to $\hat{F}_n$ is typically approximated using simulation. Such simulation involves generating random samples from $\hat{F}_n$, and it is here that the necessity of resampling emerges. The empirical distribution function $\hat{F}_n$ is equivalent to a cumulative distribution function from a discrete probability distribution that places probability $\frac{1}{n}$ on each of the observed sample values y_i. Sampling from $\hat{F}_n$ can therefore be achieved by sampling at random from the observed sample values. In particular, a new sample generated from the original sample using $\hat{F}_n$, can be generated by taking n observations at random with replacement from the original sample values $y_1, \ldots, y_n$. This means that the new sample will only include values that occurred in the original sample. Furthermore, each value in the original sample may be either present or absent from the new sample, and if it is present it may occur once or more than once.

Using the above resampling process, bootstrapping is implemented by generating B new samples, each of which is called a **replicate sample**, and all of which are generated as above by sampling with replacement from the original sample. For the jth replicate sample a **replicate estimate** $\hat{\theta}_j$ is computed, leading to a total of B replicate estimates. We then use these replicate estimates to obtain information about the sampling distribution corresponding to $\hat{\theta}$. In particular, a histogram of the B replicate estimates $\hat{\theta}_1, \ldots, \hat{\theta}_B$ provides a display of the shape of the sampling distribution which could be used to assess, for example, approximate normality. Furthermore, the sample variance of the replicate estimates provides an estimate of the variance of the sampling distribution. This means that a bootstrap estimate of standard error is

$$\text{se}(\hat{\theta}) = \sqrt{\frac{1}{B-1} \sum_{j=1}^{B} \left(\hat{\theta}_j - \bar{\theta}\right)^2}$$

where $\bar{\theta}$ is the mean of the B replicate estimates. Confidence interval estimation is also possible, the simplest method being the so-called **percentile method**. This involves simply using the relevant percentiles of the replicate estimates as the end-points of the confidence interval. That is, a $(1-2\alpha)100\%$ bootstrap confidence interval is $\left(\hat{\theta}_{(B\alpha)}, \hat{\theta}_{(B-B\alpha)}\right)$, where $\hat{\theta}_{(j)}$ is the jth largest replicate estimate. For example, if $B = 1000$ then a 95% bootstrap confidence interval is $\left(\hat{\theta}_{(25)}, \hat{\theta}_{(975)}\right)$, using the percentile method.

An important consideration when using bootstrapping is the choice of B, the number of bootstrap replicates. There is no simple answer to the question of how many replicates to use, and generally speaking it is best to have as many as is feasible given the available computational resources. For confidence intervals, values of at least $B = 1000$ are typical in practice, whereas for standard errors B can smaller, perhaps $B = 200$. It is also important to bear in mind that the choice of B determines the accuracy with which the sampling distribution is estimated, but it has no effect on the sampling distribution itself. That is, choosing a larger B does not allow more information to be extracted from the sample, it just helps to minimise random fluctuations that may occur as a result of the resampling process. Of course, with B taking values as large as 1000 or more, bootstrapping can be a rather computer-intensive process.

The theoretical properties of bootstrap estimates have been well studied and generally provide a strong theoretical basis for using bootstrapping. These theoretical studies have led to many variants of the standard bootstrap described above, and it is important to be aware that such variants exist, even if a more complete study of bootstrapping procedures is beyond our scope in this book. Interested readers are referred to texts such as Efron and Tibshirani (1993) and Davison and Hinkley (1997).

One variant of the standard bootstrap is to use a different sample estimate of F other than the empirical distribution function $\hat{F}_n(y)$. For example, F can be estimated from the sample using a parametric model with maximum likelihood estimation, and resampling carried out from this parametric estimate rather than from the non-parametric estimate $\hat{F}_n(y)$. This leads to the terms **parametric bootstrap** and **non-parametric bootstrap** to distinguish the two approaches. Other variants aim to improve the properties of bootstrap estimates, or to extend bootstrapping to more complex inferential contexts such as regression analysis. For example, in certain circumstances the standard bootstrap procedure can be biased, in the sense that $\bar{\theta} \neq \hat{\theta}$ so that the bootstrap sampling distribution is not centred at the estimate $\hat{\theta}$. A modification of the standard bootstrap to address this is called the **bias-corrected bootstrap**, which essentially involves an adjustment of the bootstrap sampling distribution and the associated confidence intervals, according to the magnitude of the **bootstrap bias**, $\bar{\theta} - \hat{\theta}$. Importantly, however, such variants are based on resampling concepts similar to those used for the standard bootstrap described above, which are illustrated in the following example.

Example 8.5 In Section 2.10 and Example 8.3 we considered a sample of $n = 100$ cholesterol levels, including standard error estimation and the construction of 95% confidence intervals based on the sample mean $\bar{y}$ and the sample median m. In particular, we used confidence intervals based on normal approximations to the sampling

TABLE 8.3

Comparison of bootstrap and normal 95% confidence intervals (CI) and
standard errors for the cholesterol example with two different sample sizes

	Bootstrap		Normal	
	$n = 20$	$n = 100$	$n = 20$	$n = 100$
mean estimate	5.25	5.26	5.25	5.26
median estimate	5.15	5.25	5.15	5.25
mean standard error	0.15	0.069	0.16	0.069
median standard error	0.14	0.086	0.20	0.087
mean CI	4.95–5.55	5.13–5.40	4.94–5.56	5.12–5.40
median CI	4.96–5.53	5.11–5.41	4.77–5.53	5.08–5.42

distributions, namely,

$$\bar{y} \pm 1.96 \frac{s_{n-1}}{\sqrt{n}} \quad \text{and} \quad m \pm 1.96 s_{n-1} \sqrt{\frac{\pi}{2n}}.$$

Bootstrapping provides an alternative method to construct these confidence intervals. We will conduct a bootstrap analysis using the full sample of $n = 100$ cholesterol levels, as well as a reduced sample of the first $n = 20$ observations. This allows us to assess the behaviour of the various interval estimates in both smaller and larger sample sizes.

In order to implement bootstrapping for these two samples, we need to take B replicate samples of size $n = 100$ or $n = 20$, with replacement from the original sample values. We then need to calculate the sample mean and sample median for each of these replicate samples, and these are our B replicate estimates. This process leads to four sets of replicate estimates, corresponding to the two sample sizes and the two estimates, mean and median. Figure 8.4 displays the results of these bootstrap analyses, using $B = 10,000$ replicates in each case. The four histograms in Figure 8.4 show the shape of the sampling distribution in each case. It can be seen that the sampling distribution of the mean seems to be approximately normal for both sample sizes, whereas for the median there seems to be some non-normality, particularly for the smaller sample size.

The bootstrap replicates in Figure 8.4 yield 95% confidence intervals using the percentile method, displayed in Table 8.3. Also displayed are bootstrap estimates of standard error, along with the results obtained using the normal approximation. It is seen in Table 8.3 that the bootstrap confidence intervals are in close agreement with the normal confidence intervals based on the sample mean, for both samples sizes. The same is true for the sample median with the larger sample size, but there is a large difference for the smaller sample size. In this case, the normal approximation is unable to accommodate the pronounced skewness of the sampling distribution, whereas the bootstrap sampling distribution is able to produce an asymmetric confidence interval that does reflect this skewness.

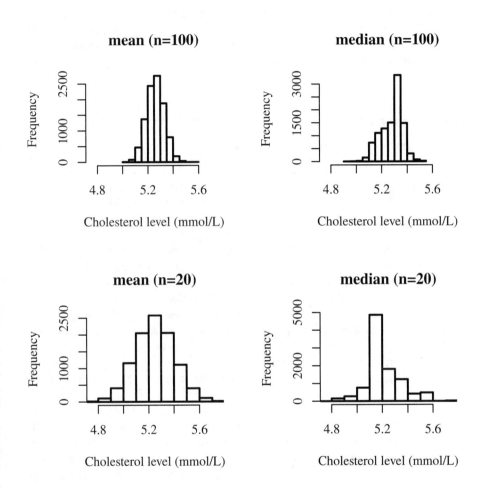

FIGURE 8.4
Histograms of 10,000 bootstrap replicates of the sample mean and sample median for the cholesterol example discussed in Example 8.3

The above results suggest that in small samples the bootstrap confidence interval based on the sample median is preferable to a confidence interval based on the normal approximation. However, it should be noted that although we have found a difference between the two methods in small samples, we have not actually justified that the bootstrap confidence interval is more accurate. One way to do this is to conduct a simulation study in which the coverage probability of the bootstrap confidence interval is compared with the coverage probability of the normal confidence interval. If this were undertaken in the present context it would show that the bootstrap confidence interval is indeed more accurate.

8.4   Further resampling methods

Random sampling with replacement from an observed sample is not the only way to undertake resampling. Indeed, some approaches to resampling do not involve simulation at all, but instead rely on deterministic schemes for generating new samples from the original sample. In this section we touch on some other resampling-based inference methods that are distinct from bootstrapping.

An historically important alternative to bootstrapping is called **jackknifing**, which was one of the first resampling methods to be proposed. Jackknifing is a very similar resampling method to bootstrapping, but the replicate samples are generated using a non-random, or deterministic, process. In particular, when undertaking jackknifing we generate new samples from the original sample by simply leaving out observations. The most common approach is the leave-one-out approach, which means that we generate a new sample by leaving out one observation from the original sample. In a sample of n observations there are n ways to leave one observation out, so jackknifing is usually applied to these n replicate samples which are each of size $n - 1$. Similarly to bootstrapping, this leads to n replicate estimates $\hat{\theta}_1, \ldots, \hat{\theta}_n$, with mean $\overline{\theta}$. Other than the fact that the replicate samples have been obtained differently, jackknife estimates of variability and bias are obtained in the same way as the corresponding bootstrap estimates. Thus, a jackknife estimate of standard error is obtained by calculating the standard deviation of the $\hat{\theta}_i$ estimates, and a jackknife estimate of bias is obtained by calculating $\overline{\theta} - \hat{\theta}$. Generalisations of this process are also possible based on leaving out more than one observation, which is called the leave-k-out approach. Although there is a similarity between bootstrapping and jackknifing, bootstrapping has some theoretical advantages over jackknifing and tends to be more informative, particularly because it yields more detailed information about the full sampling distribution, as depicted in Figure 8.4. For these reasons, bootstrapping is more commonly used in practice.

Another deterministic method for undertaking resampling is by permuting the original sample to obtain a new sample. This approach is particularly useful for two-sample problems where we want to test a null hypothesis involving equality between two groups. In this context, a new sample can be generated by simply permuting the

TABLE 8.4

Permutation samples for four observations divided into two groups and the permutation sampling distribution for the rank-sum test statistic in group 1

observation rank	group	group permutations				
1	1	1	2	2	1	2
2	2	1	1	1	2	2
3	1	2	1	2	2	1
4	2	2	2	1	1	1
t_{RS}	4	3	5	6	5	7
$\Pr(T_{RS} \leq t_{RS})$	$\frac{1}{3}$	$\frac{1}{6}$	$\frac{2}{3}$	$\frac{5}{6}$	$\frac{2}{3}$	1

group indicators. If the null hypothesis is true, that is, if the two groups have the same distribution, then the value of the test statistic in the permuted sample will have the same distribution as the value in the original sample. Thus, by enumerating all possible permuted samples and computing the test statistic in each sample, we obtain an estimate of the sampling distribution of test statistic under the null hypothesis. The value of the test statistic in the original sample can then be compared with this sampling distribution to obtain a *P*-value. This type of resampling yields a general class of tests called **permutation tests**.

Permutation tests require us to first choose a test statistic that is appropriate for the context. Having chosen the test statistic, permutation resampling provides a general method for non-parametrically estimating the sampling distribution of the test statistic under the null hypothesis. To illustrate this process, consider the rank-sum test statistic that was used in the Wilcoxon rank-sum test. Table 8.4 provides all of the possible permutation samples for a simple example of two groups each with two observations. In this case there are six possible permutations of the group indicators, including the original grouping, and the rank-sum associated with group 1 has been calculated for each sample. By assigning probability $\frac{1}{6}$ to each permutation we obtain a non-parametric estimate of the sampling distribution of the rank-sum statistic under the null hypothesis. The observed value of the rank-sum statistic in Table 8.4 is 4, with $\Pr(T_{RS} \leq 4) = \frac{1}{3}$, which can be interpreted as a one-sided *P*-value. A two-sided *P*-value would simply be double the one-sided *P*-value. This permutation procedure can actually be shown to produce the exact sampling distribution for the Wilcoxon rank-sum test that was alluded to in Section 8.2. Thus, the Wilcoxon rank-sum test can be interpreted as a permutation test.

Although we have illustrated permutation tests using the Wilcoxon rank-sum test statistic, permutation tests are in fact a general strategy that can be used for any other test statistic. For example, we could use the same process to estimate the sampling distribution of the two-sample *t*-test statistic, by calculating this test statistic for each of the possible permutation samples. This would provide us with an alternative way of testing the null hypothesis.

While Table 8.4 has only six permutations associated with the four observations, it is important to note that when the sample size is at least moderately large, then the number of possible permutation samples will become extremely large. In practice, this means that enumerating each of the possible permutation samples is highly computer intensive. Indeed, in large samples the number of permutations may be so large that complete enumeration is computationally infeasible. Thus, although permutation methods are in principle deterministic resampling methods, in practice simulation is often used to approximate the permutation sampling distribution. This simulation involves randomly sampling, with replacement, a large number of permutation samples from among the even larger number of possible permutation samples. The estimated sampling distribution can then be constructed from these random samples in much the same way as was done for the bootstrap sampling distributions depicted in Figure 8.4.

In summary, resampling methods such as bootstrapping and permutation tests are powerful and widely applicable approaches for constructing sampling distributions of estimators and test statistics. They are computationally intensive but can provide flexible alternatives to traditional methods that use large sample likelihood theory.

Exercises

1. In Section 8.1 we considered the exact sampling distribution for the prevalence estimator P and an approximate sampling distribution based on the normal distribution.

   (a) Plot the probability function of the exact sampling distribution for P, assuming a sample size of $n = 10$ and population prevalence of $\theta = 0.5$. Repeat this for $\theta = 0.1, 0.25, 0.75$ and 0.9.

   (b) Repeat part (a) using the probability density function from the approximate normal sampling distribution.

   (c) Comment on your results from parts (a) and (b).

2. In this exercise we consider a simple illustration of Fisher's exact test. Consider again the extended example from Chapter 5, but for illustrative purposes we will now suppose that the data table given in Table 5.2 has just $n = 4$ individuals with column totals $n_0 = 2$ and $n_1 = 2$ denoting the number of individuals on monotherapy and combination therapy, respectively, and response total $x_0 + x_1 = 2$.

   (a) Show that there are 3 possible 2×2 configurations and enumerate each of these.

   (b) Using the hypergeometric probability given in Section 8.1, calculate the probability associated with each of the 2×2 configurations. Check that the probabilities sum to 1.

(c) Suppose both individuals on combination therapy experienced a response while both individuals on monotherapy did not respond. Give the *P*-value for Fisher's exact test for testing whether there is a difference in response rates between the two therapies.

3. Consider the sample of HIV viral load reductions given in Table 8.2. In Example 8.4 we considered the Wilcoxon signed-rank test for this sample. In this exercise we will consider the sign test. Let w_p be the observed number of positive observations in the sample, which can be considered the observed value of a random variable W_p.

   (a) Under the null hypothesis that the population median reduction in viral load is zero, state the distribution of W_p.

   (b) Give a large sample normal approximation to the distribution in part (a).

   (c) By comparing the observed value w_p with the sampling distribution from part (a), compute a two-sided *P*-value for testing the null hypothesis that the median reduction is zero. Compare the result with the Wilcoxon signed-rank test in Example 8.4.

   (d) Repeat part (c) using the large sample normal approximation to the sampling distribution.

   (e) Would you expect the power of the sign test to be better or worse than the power of the Wilcoxon signed-rank test? Give reasons.

   (f) State an assumption of the Wilcoxon signed-rank test that is not necessary when using the sign test.

4. Now suppose that we have viral load reductions for a second group of individuals. For the purposes of illustration, we will construct this second group of viral load reductions by multiplying each observation in Table 8.2 by 3.

   (a) Combine the two groups of observations and determine the ranks in the combined sample of 50 observations. Hence compute the observed value of T_{RS}, the sum of the ranks of the observations from the first group.

   (b) Using the normal approximation to the sampling distribution of T_{RS}, compute the *P*-value of the Wilcoxon rank-sum test for a difference in the medians from the two groups, using a two-sided alternative hypothesis.

   (c) Compare your result in part (b) with the result from a two-sample *t*-test. Which of the two test tests do you think is more appropriate for these data?

5. In this exercise we will consider bootstrapping for the sample in Table 8.2.

   (a) Compute a 95% bootstrap confidence interval for the population median viral load reduction. Use the function bootstrap in Appendix 2 with $B = 1000$ bootstrap replications.

   (b) Compare this bootstrap confidence interval with the confidence interval that would be obtained using a large sample normal approximation to the sampling distribution of the median.

(c) Plot a histogram of the B bootstrap medians. Identify the sample median and the limits of the two confidence intervals on the plot. Comment on the sampling distribution of the median and your results in part (b).

(d) Repeat parts (a) through (c) for the mean.

6. Suppose we have a sample with two groups of three observations: $(10, 12, 15)$ from group 1 and $(14, 17, 18)$ from group 2.

(a) Construct a table analogous to Table 8.4 for this sample. Including the original sample, there are 20 possible permutations.

(b) Compute the permutation sampling distribution associated with the rank-sum test statistic, by assigning probability $\frac{1}{20}$ to each possible permutation.

(c) Hence compute the P-value for this sample using a permutation test based on the rank-sum test statistic.

(d) In the above analysis we used the rank-sum test statistic. Suppose instead that we use the two-sample t-test statistic

$$\frac{\bar{x}_1 - \bar{x}_2}{\sqrt{\frac{s_1^2}{n_1} + \frac{s_2^2}{n_2}}}.$$

Calculate this test statistic for each of the 20 permutation samples. Hence compute the P-value for this sample using a permutation test based on the two-sample t-test statistic.

Appendices

Appendix 1: Common probability distributions

In this appendix we review some common probability distributions that are used in this book. The notation $F_X(x)$ denotes the cumulative distribution function, and $f_X(x)$ denotes either the probability function or the probability density function, depending on whether the distribution is discrete or continuous. For each distribution the function $f_X(x)$ is specified for x in the set of possible values for that distribution, and is interpreted to be zero otherwise.

Binomial distribution

$$X \stackrel{d}{=} \mathrm{Bin}(n, p)$$

Discrete distribution used to model the number of successes in n independent trials each having probability p of success.

$$f_X(x) = \Pr(X = x) = \frac{n!}{(n-x)!\,x!} p^x(1-p)^x \qquad x = 0, 1, \ldots, n \quad 0 \le p \le 1$$

$$\mathrm{E}(X) = np \qquad \mathrm{Var}(X) = np(1-p).$$

When n is large the binomial distribution can be approximated by a normal distribution $\mathrm{N}(np, np(1-p))$. When n is large and p is small, the binomial distribution can be approximated by a Poisson distribution $\mathrm{Pois}(np)$.

Poisson distribution

$$X \stackrel{d}{=} \mathrm{Pois}(\lambda)$$

Discrete distribution used to model counts, often the number of independent events occurring in an interval of time.

$$f_X(x) = \Pr(X = x) = \frac{\lambda^x e^{-\lambda}}{x!} \qquad x = 0, 1, 2, \ldots \quad \lambda > 0$$

$$\mathrm{E}(X) = \lambda \qquad \mathrm{Var}(X) = \lambda.$$

When λ is large, the Poisson distribution can be approximated by a normal distribution $\mathrm{N}(\lambda, \lambda)$. The sum of independent Poisson random variables has a Poisson distribution, with parameter equal to the sum of the parameters from the individual distributions.

Geometric distribution

$$X \stackrel{d}{=} G(p)$$

Discrete distribution used to model the number of trials until the first success, where each trial is independent and has success probability p.

$$f_X(x) = \Pr(X = x) = p(1-p)^{x-1} \qquad x = 1,2,\ldots \quad 0 < p \le 1$$

$$E(X) = \frac{1}{p} \qquad \text{Var}(X) = \frac{1-p}{p^2}.$$

Negative binomial distribution

$$X \stackrel{d}{=} NB(r,p)$$

Discrete distribution used to model the number of trials until r successes, where each trial is independent and has success probability p.

$$f_X(x) = \Pr(X = x) = \frac{(x-1)!}{(r-1)!(x-r)!} p^r(1-p)^{x-r} \qquad x = r,r+1,\ldots \quad 0 < p \le 1$$

$$E(X) = \frac{r}{p} \qquad \text{Var}(X) = \frac{r(1-p)}{p^2}.$$

The $NB(1,p)$ distribution is equivalent to the $G(p)$ distribution. The sum of r independent random variables each with a $G(p)$ distribution has a $NB(r,p)$ distribution.

Hypergeometric distribution

$$X \stackrel{d}{=} Hg(n,R,N)$$

Discrete distribution used to model the number of individuals with a particular trait in a sample of n individuals taken at random without replacement from a population of N individuals, R of whom have the particular trait. The parameters n, R and N are all non-negative integers with $n \le N$ and $R \le N$.

$$f_X(x) = \Pr(X = x) = \frac{\binom{R}{x}\binom{N-R}{n-x}}{\binom{N}{n}} \qquad x = \max(0, n+R-N), \ldots, \min(n,R)$$

$$E(X) = \frac{nR}{N} \qquad \text{Var}(X) = \frac{nR(N-R)(N-n)}{N^2(N-1)}.$$

For large R and N, the $Hg(n,R,N)$ distribution is approximately a $Bin(n,p)$ distribution with $p = R/N$, meaning that in large populations, sampling without replacement can be approximated by sampling with replacement.

Normal distribution

$$X \stackrel{d}{=} N(\mu, \sigma^2)$$

Continuous distribution used to model quantities that are symmetrically distributed around their mean, and may possibly be negative or positive.

$$f_X(x) = \frac{1}{\sigma\sqrt{2\pi}} \exp\left\{-\frac{(x-\mu)^2}{2\sigma^2}\right\} \qquad x \in (-\infty, \infty) \quad \mu \in (-\infty, \infty) \quad \sigma > 0$$

$$E(X) = \mu \qquad \text{Var}(X) = \sigma^2.$$

The $N(0, 1)$ distribution is referred to as the standard normal distribution. The cumulative distribution function of the standard normal distribution, denoted

$$\Phi(x) = \frac{1}{\sqrt{2\pi}} \int_{-\infty}^{x} \exp\left\{-\frac{u^2}{2}\right\} du \qquad x \in (-\infty, \infty)$$

does not have an explicit form, but can be calculated using tables and in most statistical software packages. For any normal distribution, the cumulative distribution function can be calculated using the relationship

$$F_X(x) = \Phi\left(\frac{x-\mu}{\sigma}\right) \qquad x \in (-\infty, \infty).$$

Due to the Central Limit Theorem, the mean or sum of a large number of independent and identically distributed random variables has an approximate normal distribution.

Exponential distribution

$$X \stackrel{d}{=} \text{Exp}(\lambda)$$

Continuous distribution for positive quantities, primarily used to model time variables, such as the time between two events.

$$f_X(x) = \lambda e^{-\lambda x} \qquad x \geq 0 \quad \lambda > 0$$

$$F_X(x) = \begin{cases} 1 - e^{-\lambda x} & x \geq 0 \\ 0 & x < 0 \end{cases}$$

$$E(X) = \frac{1}{\lambda} \qquad \text{Var}(X) = \frac{1}{\lambda^2}.$$

Gamma distribution

$$X \stackrel{d}{=} \text{Gamma}(\alpha, \beta)$$

Continuous distribution for positive quantities, commonly used in Bayesian inference to model the prior distribution of a positive parameter, such as λ in the Poisson distribution.

$$f_X(x) = \frac{\beta^\alpha x^{\alpha-1} e^{-\beta x}}{\Gamma(\alpha)} \qquad x > 0 \quad \alpha > 0 \quad \beta > 0$$

$$E(X) = \frac{\alpha}{\beta} \qquad \mathrm{Var}(X) = \frac{\alpha}{\beta^2}$$

where $\Gamma(\alpha)$ is a special mathematical function called the gamma function, defined as

$$\Gamma(\alpha) = \int_0^\infty u^{\alpha-1} e^{-u} du$$
$$= (\alpha - 1)! \quad \text{if } \alpha \text{ is a positive integer.}$$

The gamma probability density function can take a wide variety of shapes on the interval $(0, \infty)$. If $\alpha > 1$ then the distribution is unimodal inside the interval $(0, \infty)$ with mode

$$\mathrm{mode}(X) = \frac{\alpha - 1}{\beta}.$$

When α is large then the gamma distribution can be approximated by a normal distribution. The Gamma$(1, \beta)$ distribution is equivalent to the Exp(β) distribution. The sum of α independent Exp(β) random variables has a Gamma(α, β) distribution.

Uniform distribution

$$X \overset{d}{=} \mathrm{Uniform}(a, b)$$

Continuous distribution used to model random variables that are equally likely to fall into any interval of a given length within the interval $[a, b]$. In other words, the random variable is distributed evenly within the interval $[a, b]$.

$$f_X(x) = \frac{1}{b - a} \qquad -\infty < a \leq x \leq b < \infty$$

$$F_X(x) = \begin{cases} 0 & x < 0 \\ \frac{x}{b-a} & 0 \leq x \leq 1 \\ 1 & x > 1 \end{cases}$$

$$E(X) = \frac{a + b}{2} \qquad \mathrm{Var}(X) = \frac{(b - a)^2}{12}.$$

The most common uniform distribution is Uniform$(0, 1)$, in which case $f_X(x) = 1$ and $F_X(x) = x$ for $0 \leq x \leq 1$.

Beta distribution

$$X \overset{d}{=} \mathrm{Beta}(\alpha, \beta)$$

Continuous distribution defined on the interval $[0, 1]$, commonly used in Bayesian inference to model the prior distribution of a parameter that is a probability, such as p in the binomial distribution.

$$f_X(x) = \frac{x^{\alpha-1}(1 - x)^{\beta-1}}{B(\alpha, \beta)} \qquad 0 \leq x \leq 1 \quad \alpha > 0 \quad \beta > 0$$

$$E(X) = \frac{\alpha}{\alpha + \beta} \qquad Var(X) = \frac{\alpha\beta}{(\alpha+\beta)^2(\alpha+\beta+1)}$$

where $B(\alpha,\beta)$ is a special mathematical function called the beta function, which can be expressed in terms of the gamma function describe above

$$B(\alpha,\beta) = \int_0^1 x^{\alpha-1}(1-x)^{\beta-1}dx = \frac{\Gamma(\alpha)\Gamma(\beta)}{\Gamma(\alpha+\beta)}.$$

The beta probability density function can take a wide variety of shapes on the interval $[0,1]$. If $\alpha > 1$ and $\beta > 1$ then the distribution is unimodal inside the interval $(0,1)$ with mode

$$mode(X) = \frac{\alpha - 1}{\alpha + \beta - 2}.$$

When α and β are both large then the beta distribution can be approximated by a normal distribution. The Beta$(1,1)$ distribution is equivalent to the Uniform$(0,1)$ distribution.

$t-$**distribution**

$$X \stackrel{d}{=} t_\nu$$

Continuous distribution symmetric around zero but with wider tails, or more variability, than the standard normal distribution.

$$f_X(x) = \left[\sqrt{\nu}B\left(\frac{1}{2},\frac{\nu}{2}\right)\right]^{-1}\left[1 + \frac{x^2}{\nu}\right]^{-(\nu+1)/2} \qquad x \in (-\infty,\infty) \quad \nu > 0$$

where $B(\alpha,\beta)$ is the beta function discussed above. Although the probability density function is defined for $\nu > 0$, the mean and variance are finite only for $\nu > 1$ and $\nu > 2$, respectively,

$$E(X) = 0 \qquad Var(X) = \frac{\nu}{\nu - 2}.$$

The parameter ν is called the degrees of freedom and is usually an integer. As $\nu \to \infty$ the t_ν distribution converges to the standard normal distribution. The primary use is as the sampling distribution of the sample mean $\overline{X}$ of a sample of n independent $N(\mu,\sigma^2)$ random variables, after standardisation using the sample variance. In particular,

$$\frac{\overline{X} - \mu}{S_{n-1}/\sqrt{n}} \stackrel{d}{=} t_{n-1}$$

where S_{n-1}^2 is the sample variance dividing by $n-1$. The cumulative distribution function does not have an explicit form, but can be calculated using tables and in most statistical software packages.

χ^2−distribution

$$X \overset{d}{=} \chi^2(v)$$

Continuous distribution for positive quantities, primarily used in hypothesis testing.

$$f_X(x) = \frac{x^{(v-2)/2}e^{-x/2}}{2^{v/2}\Gamma(v/2)} \qquad x \geq 0 \quad v > 0$$

$$E(X) = v \qquad \text{Var}(X) = 2v$$

where $\Gamma(x)$ is the gamma function discussed above. The parameter v is called the degrees of freedom and is usually an integer. If X has a standard normal distribution then X^2 has a $\chi^2(1)$ distribution. If $X_1,\ldots,X_v$ are independent standard normal random variables then $X_1^2 + \cdots + X_v^2$ has a $\chi^2(v)$ distribution. If X_1 and X_2 are independent random variables with $\chi^2(v_1)$ and $\chi^2(v_2)$ distributions, respectively, then $X_1 + X_2$ has a $\chi^2(v_1 + v_2)$ distribution. The cumulative distribution function does not have an explicit form, but can be calculated using tables and in most statistical software packages.

F−distribution

$$X \overset{d}{=} F_{m,n}$$

Continuous distribution for positive quantities, primarily used in hypothesis testing.

$$f_X(x) = \left[xB\left(\frac{m}{2},\frac{n}{2}\right) \right]^{-1} \sqrt{\frac{(mx)^m n^n}{(mx+n)^{m+n}}} \qquad x \geq 0 \quad m > 0 \quad n > 0$$

where $B(\alpha,\beta)$ is the beta function discussed above. Although the probability density function is defined for $m > 0$ and $n > 0$, the mean and variance are finite only for $n > 2$ and $n > 4$, respectively,

$$E(X) = \frac{n}{n-2} \qquad \text{Var}(X) = \frac{2n^2(m+n-2)}{m(n-2)^2(n-4)}.$$

The parameters m and n are called the degrees of freedom and are usually integers. If $M \overset{d}{=} \chi^2(m)$ and $N \overset{d}{=} \chi^2(n)$, independently, then

$$\frac{M/m}{N/n} \overset{d}{=} F_{m,n}.$$

The square of a random variable with a t_v distribution has a $F_{1,v}$ distribution. The cumulative distribution function does not have an explicit form, but can be calculated using tables and in most statistical software packages.

Multivariate normal distribution

$$\mathbf{X} \stackrel{d}{=} N_k(\mu, \Sigma)$$

Generalisation of the normal distribution, giving the joint distribution of a $k \times 1$ vector of random variables $\mathbf{X} = (X_1, \ldots, X_k)^{\mathrm{T}}$. The distribution has many uses, but its main use in this book is as the sampling distribution of an estimator of a k-dimensional parameter. The vector $\mu = (\mu_1, \ldots, \mu_k)^{\mathrm{T}}$ is called the mean vector and can be any vector in $\mathfrak{R}^k$. The $k \times k$ matrix Σ is called the variance-covariance matrix and must be a non-negative definite matrix. Using the notation σ_{ij}^2 for the (i, j) element of Σ

$$E(X_i) = \mu_i \qquad \mathrm{Var}(X_i) = \sigma_{ii}^2 \qquad \mathrm{Cov}(X_i, X_j) = \sigma_{ij}^2.$$

The joint probability density function is

$$f_{\mathbf{X}}(\mathbf{x}) = \left[(2\pi)^k \det(\Sigma)\right]^{-\frac{1}{2}} \exp\left\{-\frac{1}{2}(\mathbf{x} - \mu)^{\mathrm{T}} \Sigma^{-1} (\mathbf{x} - \mu)\right\} \qquad \mathbf{x} \in \mathfrak{R}^k$$

where $\det(\Sigma)$ is the matrix determinant of Σ. For $k = 1$ the distribution is the normal distribution, sometimes called the univariate normal distribution. For $k = 2$ the distribution is called the bivariate normal distribution, and for $k > 2$ it is called the multivariate normal distribution. If $\mathbf{X}$ has a multivariate normal distribution then each X_i has a univariate normal distribution. If $\sigma_{ij}^2 = 0$, meaning that X_i and X_j are uncorrelated, then X_i and X_j are independent.

Appendix 2: Simulation tools

Some of the chapter exercises require simulation of random samples from various probability distributions. The chapter examples and extended examples also make use of simulation. These simulations can be carried out using any software that allows simulation of random numbers from a specified probability distribution. In this appendix we provide code for some functions that can be used in the R computing environment to conduct such simulations. R is a software environment for statistical computing and graphics that is freely available for download at www.r-project.org. Also contained on the website are various guides and manuals for using R, as well as lists of books and other references that discuss R. The R environment has many functions for simulating random samples from a probability distribution. The five R functions used in the code below are:

runif(n,min,max) simulates n observations from the Uniform(a,b) distribution with $a = $ min and $b = $ max

rnorm(n,mean,sd) simulates n observations from the N(μ, σ^2) distribution with $\mu = $ mean and $\sigma = $ sd

rbinom(n,size,prob) simulates n observations from the Bin(n,p) distribution with $n = $ size and $p = $ prob

rpois(n,lambda) simulates n observations from the Pois(λ) distribution with $\lambda = $ lambda

sample(n,replace=TRUE) randomly samples with replacement from the numbers $1, \ldots, $ n which is useful in bootstrapping

These simulation functions are used below for four types of random sample functions:

prev.sim simulation of binomial prevalence samples

inc.sim simulation of Poisson incidence samples

cnorm.sim simulation of various statistics from normal and contaminated normal samples with outliers

bootstrap bootstrapping for means and medians by random sampling with replacement from a given sample

Each of these functions requires certain input parameters detailed below, and produces output that is an R list with certain components containing the simulation results, also detailed below. These results can be viewed directly or used as input to other R functions, such as the graphical functions plot and hist, and the summary functions mean, var and summary. The functions also produce plots summarising the simulation results.

R code for function `prev.sim`

Input parameters:

`Nstudies` number of studies or samples to simulate

`N` number of individuals in each sample

`P` population prevalence

Output components:

`prev` sample prevalence from each simulated sample

`CI.low` lower endpoint of the 95% confidence interval from each simulated sample

`CI.upp` upper endpoint of the 95% confidence interval from each simulated sample

`coverage` proportion of simulations in which the confidence interval covers P

R code for `prev.sim`:

```
prev.sim=function(Nstudies,N,P) {
obs=rbinom(Nstudies,N,P)
prev=obs/N
CI.upp=prev+1.96*sqrt(prev*(1-prev)/N)
CI.low=prev-1.96*sqrt(prev*(1-prev)/N)
coverage=sum((CI.low <= P)&(P <= CI.upp))/Nstudies
hist(prev,main="Prevalence estimates",xlab="prevalence")
out=list(prev=prev,CI.low=CI.low,CI.upp=CI.upp,coverage=coverage)
out
}


#----------------------------------------------------------------
# Example 1 (non-normal sampling distribution and poor coverage)
# 1000 studies of size 10 with population prevalence 0.2
#----------------------------------------------------------------
prev.10=prev.sim(1000,10,0.2)
prev.10$coverage


#----------------------------------------------------------------
# Example 2 (normal sampling distribution and good coverage)
# 1000 studies of size 1000 with population prevalence 0.2
#----------------------------------------------------------------
prev.1000=prev.sim(1000,1000,0.2)
prev.1000$coverage
```

R code for function `inc.sim`

Input parameters:

`Nstudies` number of studies or samples to simulate

`N` number of individuals in each sample

`A` average follow-up per individual

`lambda` population incidence rate

Output components:

`inc` sample incidence rate from each simulated sample

`CI.low` lower endpoint of the 95% confidence interval from each simulated sample

`CI.upp` upper endpoint of the 95% confidence interval from each simulated sample

`coverage` proportion of simulations in which the confidence interval covers `lambda`

R code for `inc.sim`:

```
inc.sim=function(Nstudies,N,A,lambda) {
F=A*N
obs=rpois(Nstudies,F*lambda)
inc=obs/F
CI.upp=inc+1.96*sqrt(inc/F)
CI.low=inc-1.96*sqrt(inc/F)
coverage=sum((CI.low <= lambda)&(lambda <= CI.upp))/Nstudies
hist(inc,main="Incidence estimates",xlab="incidence")
out=list(inc=inc,CI.low=CI.low,CI.upp=CI.upp,coverage=coverage)
out
}


#------------------------------------------------------------------
# Example 1 (non-normal sampling distribution and poor coverage)
# 1000 studies of size 10 with average follow-up 5 years and
# population incidence rate 0.02 per year
#------------------------------------------------------------------
inc.10=inc.sim(1000,10,5,0.02)
inc.10$coverage


#------------------------------------------------------------------
# Example 2 (normal sampling distribution and good coverage)
# 1000 studies of size 1000 with average follow-up 5 years and
# population incidence rate 0.02 per year
#------------------------------------------------------------------
inc.1000=inc.sim(1000,1000,5,0.02)
inc.1000$coverage
```

R code for function `cnorm.sim`

The function `cnorm.sim` simulates various statistics from normal and contaminated normal samples with outliers. If contaminated samples are simulated then a certain proportion of the observations come from a uniform distribution rather than a normal distribution. The statistics simulated include the mean, median, variance and interquartile range, as well as *P*-values from certain hypothesis tests.

Input parameters:

`Nstudies` number of studies or samples to simulate

`N` number of individuals in each sample

`mu` population mean

`sigma` population standard deviation

`k` proportion of observations that are outliers ($k = 0$ means no outliers)

`con.low` lower limit of the uniform outlier distribution

`con.upp` upper limit of the uniform outlier distribution

`alpha` significance level for the *t*-test and signed rank test

Output components:

`means` sample mean from each simulated sample

`meds` sample median from each simulated sample

`vars` sample variance from each simulated sample

`IQRs` sample interquartile range from each simulated sample

`pt` *P*-value from a one-sample *t*-test of $mu = 0$

`pt` *P*-value from a one-sample signed rank test of $mu = 0$

`pt.sig` proportion of samples where the *t*-test was significant

`pw.sig` proportion of samples where the signed rank test was significant

R code for `cnorm.sim`:

```
cnorm.sim=
function(Nstudies,N,mu,sigma,k=0,con.low=0,con.upp=0,alpha=0.05) {
out=list(means=0,meds=0,vars=0,IQRs=0,pt=0,pw=0,pt.sig=0,pw.sig=0)
for (i in 1:Nstudies) {
obsi=rnorm(N,mu,sigma)
if ((k>0)&(k<1)) {
randi=runif(N)
coni=runif(N,con.low,con.upp)
obsi[randi<=k]=coni[randi<=k]
}
out$means[i]=mean(obsi)
out$meds[i]=median(obsi)
out$vars[i]=var(obsi)
out$IQRs[i]=IQR(obsi)
out$pt[i]=t.test(obsi)$p.value
out$pw[i]=wilcox.test(obsi)$p.value
}
out$pt.sig=sum(out$pt<=alpha)/Nstudies
out$pw.sig=sum(out$pw<=alpha)/Nstudies
out}
#----------------------------------------------------------------
# Example 1 (efficiency of sample median relative to mean)
# 1000 studies of size 100 from standard normal distribution
# with either no outliers or 10% outliers from Uniform(-10,10)
#----------------------------------------------------------------
cnorm0=cnorm.sim(1000,100,0,1,k=0)
var(cnorm0$means)/var(cnorm0$meds)
cnorm10=cnorm.sim(1000,100,0,1,k=0.1,-10,10)
var(cnorm10$means)/var(cnorm10$meds)
#----------------------------------------------------------------
# Example 2 (coverage probability of 95% confidence interval)
# 1000 studies of size 100 from standard normal distribution
#----------------------------------------------------------------
cnorm01=cnorm.sim(1000,100,0,1,k=0)
CI.lower=cnorm01$means - 1.96*sqrt(cnorm01$vars/100)
CI.upper=cnorm01$means + 1.96*sqrt(cnorm01$vars/100)
coverage=sum( (CI.lower <= 0) & (CI.upper >= 0) )/1000
#----------------------------------------------------------------
# Example 3 (power of t-test and signed rank test)
# 1000 studies of size 100 from N(.2,1) distribution
#----------------------------------------------------------------
cnorm.2=cnorm.sim(1000,100,0.2,1,k=0)
cnorm.2$pt.sig
cnorm.2$pw.sig
```

R code for function `bootstrap`

The function `bootstrap` carries out simple bootstrapping of means and medians from a given sample. It produces a confidence interval using the percentile method and a standard error, along with the bootstrap replications. The code could easily be extended to provide bootstrapping of estimates other than the mean and median.

Input parameters:

`samp` sample of observations for which bootstrapping is required

`B` number of bootstrap replications

`estimate` the type of estimate to bootstrap, either `"mean"` or `"median"`

`confidence` confidence level for the confidence interval

Output components:

`reps` collection of bootstrap replications of the mean or median

`SE` standard error estimate

`CI` confidence interval

R code for `bootstrap`:

```
#----------------------------------------------
# Function bootstrap for simple bootstrapping
#----------------------------------------------

bootstrap=function(samp,B=1000,estimate="mean",confidence=0.95) {
out=list(reps=0,SE=0,CI=0)
reps=0
n=length(samp)
for (i in 1:B) {
rep=sample(n,replace=TRUE)
if (estimate=="mean") reps[i]=mean(samp[rep])
if (estimate=="median") reps[i]=median(samp[rep])
}
low=floor(B*(1-confidence)/2)
upp=ceiling(B*(1-(1-confidence)/2))
SE=sqrt(var(reps))
CI=sort(reps)[c(low,upp)]
out$reps=reps
out$SE=SE
out$CI=CI
out
}
```

```
#----------------------------------------------------------------
# Example
# Sample of size 25 is generated from the N(0,1) distribution
# Bootstrapping of the mean with B=1000
#----------------------------------------------------------------

samp=rnorm(25)
boot.25=bootstrap(samp,B=1000,estimate="mean")
boot.25$CI # 95% confidence interval
boot.25$SE # standard error
hist(boot.25$reps) # sampling distribution
```

Appendix 3: Further reading

The purpose of this book is to provide a conceptual and theoretical foundation on which to approach more advanced topics in biostatistical methodology. As the Preface states, the book presents the principles of statistical inference from a biostatistical perspective. The presentation therefore sits somewhere between books providing a compendium of biostatistical methods and texts for a traditional course on mathematical statistics. There are many books that provide further reading at each end of this spectrum. Texts providing a broad overview of basic and moderately advanced biostatistical methods include the books by Armitage et al. (2002), Rosner (2010), Lachin (2010) and Clayton and Hills (1993). Texts providing the basis of a traditional graduate course in mathematical statistics include Casella and Berger (2001), Hogg et al. (2013), Wackerly et al. (2008) and Azzalini (1996). For the more advanced reader, the books by Lehmann and Casella (1998) and Lehmann and Romano (2005) provide a definitive treatment of the theory of statistical estimation and testing, while the book by Cox and Hinkley (1974) is a classic text in the field.

Our discussion of the interpretations of probability and the presentation of both frequentist and Bayesian methods raises issues in the foundations of statistical inference. The book by Cox (2006) provides an in-depth discussion of foundational issues while the article by Bayarri and Berger (2004) provides a comparative discussion of frequentist and Bayesian inference. Books presenting a detailed treatment of the concept of likelihood and likelihood-based methods include Edwards (1992) and Royall (1997), while the book by Young and Smith (2005) also provides an overview of the different approaches to statistical inference.

We have discussed inference principles in the context of relatively basic models, for the purpose of providing the theoretical underpinnings for core analysis methodologies. Books that have sections or chapters presenting likelihood-based motivation for more advanced models, such as linear and generalised linear models, include Kleinbaum et al. (2008), Dobson and Barnett (2008) and McCullagh and Nelder (1989), while the books by Gelman et al. (2013) and Lee (2012) present more advanced Bayesian analysis methodologies, including hierarchical models. Likewise, our treatment of the further inference topics described in Chapter 8 was limited to a brief introduction. General texts such as Armitage et al. (2002), Wackerly et al. (2008) and Hogg et al. (2013) have sections or chapters providing introductions to the topics discussed in Chapter 8, while the books by Lehmann (2006), Gibbons and Chakraborti (2011), Efron and Tibshirani (1993) and Davison and Hinkley (1997) provide more detailed presentations of these topics.

Bibliography

Armitage, P., Berry, G., and Matthews, J. (2002). *Statistical Methods in Medical Research*. Blackwell Science, Oxford, UK, fourth edition.

Azzalini, A. (1996). *Statistical Inference: Based on the Likelihood*. Chapman & Hall, London, UK.

Bayarri, M. and Berger, J. (2004). The interplay between Bayesian and frequentist analysis. *Statistical Science*, 19:58–80.

Carlin, B. and Louis, T. (2000). *Bayes and Empirical Bayes Methods for Data Analysis*. Chapman & Hall/CRC, Boca Raton, FL, USA, second edition.

Casella, G. and Berger, R. (2001). *Statistical Inference*. Brooks/Cole, Boston, MA, USA, second edition.

Clayton, D. and Hills, M. (1993). *Statistical Models in Epidemiology*. Oxford University Press, Oxford, UK.

Cox, D. (2006). *Principles of Statistical Inference*. Cambridge University Press, Cambridge, UK.

Cox, D. and Hinkley, D. (1974). *Theoretical Statistics*. Chapman & Hall, London, UK.

Davison, A. and Hinkley, D. (1997). *Bootstrap Methods and their Application*. Cambridge University Press, Cambridge, UK.

Dobson, A. and Barnett, A. (2008). *An Introduction to Generalized Linear Models*. Chapman & Hall/CRC, Boca Raton, FL, USA, third edition.

Edwards, A. (1992). *Likelihood*. Johns Hopkins University Press, Baltimore, USA, expanded edition.

Efron, B. and Tibshirani, T. (1993). *An Introduction to the Bootstrap*. Chapman & Hall, London, UK.

Gelman, A., Carlin, J., Stern, H., Dunson, D., Vehtari, A., and Rubin, D. (2013). *Bayesian Data Analysis*. Chapman & Hall/CRC, Boca Raton, FL, USA, third edition.

Gibbons, J. and Chakraborti, S. (2011). *Nonparametric Statistical Inference*. Chapman & Hall/CRC, Boca Raton, FL, USA, fifth edition.

Hogg, R., McKean, J., and Craig, A. (2013). *Introduction to Mathematical Statistics.* Pearson Education, Boston, MA, USA, seventh edition.

Kleinbaum, D., Kupper, L., Nizam, A., and Muller, K. (2008). *Applied Regression Analysis and Other Multivariable Methods.* Thomson Brooks/Cole, Belmont, CA, USA, fourth edition.

Lachin, J. (2010). *Biostatistical Methods: The Assessment of Relative Risks.* John Wiley & Sons, Hoboken, NJ, USA, second edition.

Lee, P. (2012). *Bayesian Statistics: An Introduction.* John Wiley & Sons, Hoboken, NJ, USA, fourth edition.

Lehmann, E. (2006). *Nonparametrics: Statistical Methods Based on Ranks.* Springer, New York, NY, USA, revised edition.

Lehmann, E. and Casella, G. (1998). *Theory of Point Estimation.* Springer, New York, NY, USA, second edition.

Lehmann, E. and Romano, J. (2005). *Testing Statistical Hypothesis.* Springer, New York, NY, USA, third edition.

McCullagh, P. and Nelder, J. (1989). *Generalized Linear Models.* Chapman & Hall, London, UK, second edition.

Rosner, B. (2010). *Fundamentals of Biostatistics.* Cengage Learning, Boston, MA, USA, seventh edition.

Royall, R. (1997). *Statistical Evidence: A Likelihood Paradigm.* Chapman & Hall, London, UK.

Wackerly, D., Mendenhall, W., and Scheaffer, R. (2008). *Mathematical Statistics with Applications.* Thomson Brooks/Cole, Belmont, CA, USA, seventh edition.

Young, G. and Smith, R. (2005). *Essentials of Statistical Inference.* Cambridge University Press, Cambridge, UK.

Index